HERBAL
WISDOM

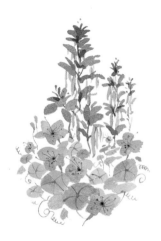

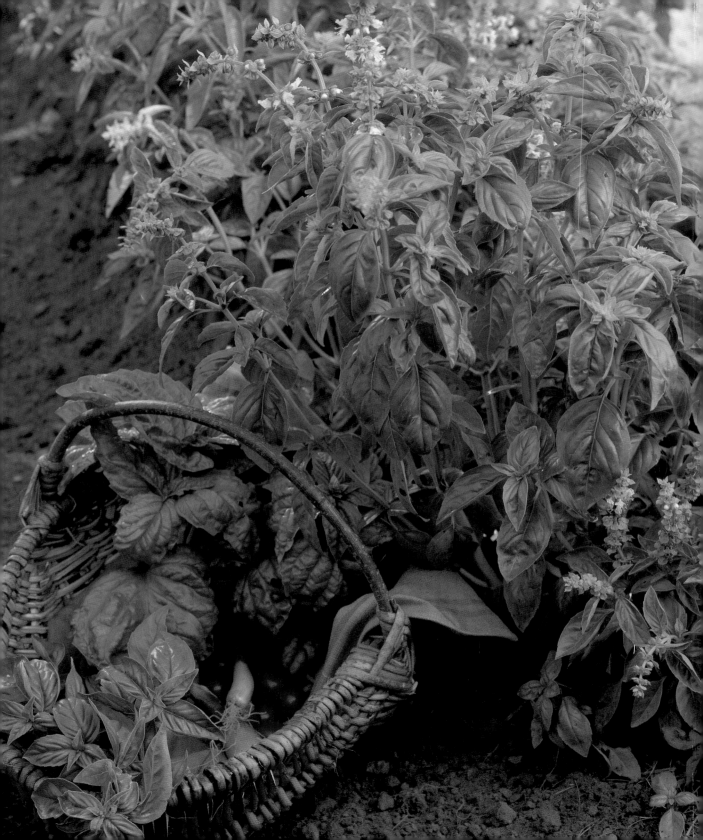

HERBAL
WISDOM

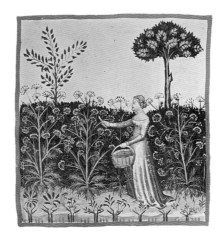

R O N I   J A Y

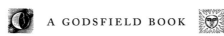
A GODSFIELD BOOK

Library of Congress Cataloging-in-Publication Data Available

10 9 8 7 6 5 4 3 2 1

Published in 1999 by Sterling Publishing Company, Inc.
387 Park Avenue South, New York, N.Y. 10016
© 1999 Godsfield Press
Text © 1999 Roni Jay

Roni Jay asserts the moral right to be identified
as the author of this work.

Distributed in Canada by Sterling Publishing
c/o Canadian Manda Group, One Atlantic Avenue, Suite 105
Toronto, Ontario, Canada M6K 3E7
Distributed in Australia by Capricorn Link (Australia) Pty Ltd
P O. Box 6651, Baulkham Hills, Business Centre, NSW 2153, Australia

Printed and bound in Hong Kong

ISBN 0-8069-7070-7

The publishers wish to thank the following for the use of pictures:

The Bridgeman Art Library pp / Markisches Museum, Berlin, Germany 10-11bc /
National Gallery of Scotland, Edinburgh 59tl / Palazzo Ducale, Mantua, Italy /
Private Collection 22b, 27t / The Stapleton Collection 6cr, 56r;
Liz Eddison pp 7br, 10bl, 18tr, 19b, 24tl, 25, 31l,r, 33t, 34, 39r, 50b, 51b, 52bl, 53b,
59tr, 64l, 65tr, 67tr, 69tr, 71b, 74bl, 76b/g, 75, 78tr, 85t, 89t, 91t, 101r, 119, 122l;
e.t.Archive pp91b
The Garden Picture Library pp 14, 20-21, 23tl, 32b, 33, 35b, 38-39bc, 42c,
45t, 46bl, 48, 49t, 52r, 54-55bc, 60r, 66-67bc, 70b, 77br, 79, 84c, 90r, 92b,
94l, 100br, 103t, 105b, 106b/g, 107b, 108-109bc, 112l, 113b/g, 114l, 115r,
116-117bc, 120b, 121b/g, 122-123bc, 124-125b/g, 126-127b/g;
The Harry Smith Collection pp 30tl, 40b, 56l, 58b, 68-69bc,
80-81bc, 82b/g, 87t, 110-111bc;
Hulton Getty p 60tl;
The Stock Market pp 29t, 72br, 78br, 95b;
Tony Stone Images pp 12b, 37t, 82b, 88b, 97t, 98tl, 99b/g.

Contents

Introduction

Herbs have been used in cooking, medicine, and magic for thousands of years, and much of the wisdom of the ancients has been passed down, and added to, through the centuries.

The ancient Chinese, Persians, Hebrews, Greeks, Druids, and many others learned to derive great value from these plants, many of which were considered sacred and used in religious rituals.

It is remarkable how many of the ancient medicinal uses of herbs have been validated by modern scientific research. Some of these uses would have been discovered by trial and error, but many were ascribed to the plants because of seemingly random attributes, such as the shape of the leaves or the appearance of the flowers. Yet many (though not all) of these unscientifically attributed powers have turned out to be correct.

ABOVE *Vervain has spiky leaves and is similar in appearance to lavender.*

ABOVE *The ancient Persians were one of many civilizations to recognize the benefit of herbs.*

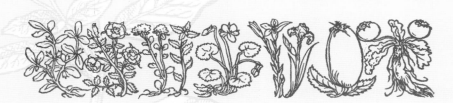

What is an Herb?

The broadest, and oldest, definition of an herb is an herbaceous plant, in other words one that disappears below ground at the end of the growing season. The word comes from the Latin herba, *which simply means grass, or green plant.*

The more popular usage of the word nowadays, however, is a plant that is useful in some way, rather than merely decorative. An herb may be used in cooking – as a flavoring or preservative – or medicine, or for its scent. Some are used cosmetically, or even as companion plants in the yard to help neighboring plants grow better. A great many herbs have multiple uses, as you will discover in this book.

Any part of a plant may be used to qualify it as an herb; not only the stems and leaves, but also the flowers or roots, or even the bark – there are some shrubs and trees that qualify as herbs, such as elder.

ABOVE *The decorative elderflower is particularly renowned for its use in wine-making.*

BELOW *Herbs have been used to enhance dishes for centuries.*

Astrology and Herbs

Each herb is associated with an astrological sign. You might expect the herbs to be linked to the signs according to the time of year they flower (or fruit). But in fact the system is much more complex than this. The ancient Greeks and Romans associated certain herbs – and other plants – with particular gods and goddesses. And many of these gods and goddesses had planets named after them: Mars, Venus, Jupiter, Saturn, and so on. As western astrology developed, the twelve zodiac signs were each ruled by one of these planets, which associated their herbs with the signs, too. So bay, for example, was sacred to the sun god Apollo. When the sun was ascribed to the sign of Leo, bay was considered to be a Leo herb. In Herbal Wisdom, *you will find each section includes a detailed description of three or four herbs that are allocated to each zodiac sign in this way.*

RIGHT
Bay has strong associations with the astrological sign of Leo, and is best harvested in late summer.

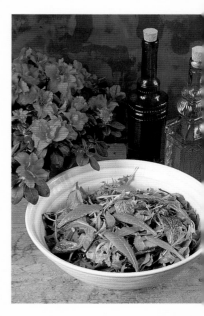

7 ☽

Astrological Herbalism

Traditionally, an astrological herbalist treated a patient by first identifying the planet that governed the part of the body in need of treatment. He then recommended the use of an herb that was associated with that planet. In the 17th century, the famous herbalist Nicholas Culpeper also advised using herbs that had the same sign as the one the patient was born under. Both of these recommendations have since lost popularity, although many herbalists still recommend that where a choice of herbs is available to treat a particular ailment, it is better to use an herb whose sign matches that of the patient or the part of the body being treated. By exploring in depth the qualities of the astrological herbs, this book gives you the opportunity to use these herbs in the broadest possible terms.

ABOVE *Nicholas Culpeper was the most famous herbalist to associate herbs and astrology.*

The Astrological Garden

The garden of a traditional herbalist, or a wise woman, was often laid out according to the zodiac. It would be set out in a wheel, with twelve "spokes" dividing the garden into twelve beds. Each of these beds would be planted with herbs belonging to one of the zodiac signs, so the signs would progress around the wheel in order.

BELOW *Respiratory problems have been traditionally treated with Pulminaria officinalis because its leaves are said to resemble spittle.*

The Doctrine of Signatures

Another important approach to herbalism in the past became known as the doctrine of signatures. The belief was that all plants were created by God to be useful, and each had its own healing properties. The illness the plant would cure was indicated by a visual clue – or signature.

Pulmonaria officinalis has large oval leaves speckled with white spots. The shape of the leaves was thought to resemble the lungs, and the white dots were spittle; so the plant was used to treat respiratory and lung diseases.

(Its common name is lungwort.) Lesser celandine has tiny tuber roots that were considered to look like hemorrhoids. So it was used to treat hemorrhoids, and as was so often the case, it acquired a common name that gave a broad hint as to its use: pilewort.

The color of an herb's flowers was sometimes considered a clue to the way it could be used medicinally. Yellow flowers, for example, were generally used in herbal treatments for illnesses such as jaundice or other liver complaints. Herbs with red flowers would be used to treat conditions of the blood and bleeding which resulted from nosebleeds, wounds, hemorrhage, and so on.

ABOVE *The color of an herb's flowers may indicate traditional medical uses.*

Sometimes the link between a plant and its attributed healing powers are quite hard to identify. The plant Echium vulgare has a brown stem that is spotted, somewhat like a snake's skin (if you have a good imagination). It also produces seeds that recall the shape of an adder's head. Therefore, according to the doctrine of signatures, the plant is an antidote to the venomous bite of the adder — and its common name is viper's bugloss.

Although the doctrine of signatures has no scientific basis that would be recognized in the modern age, it is surprising how often it has been proved to be correct. Often there is no evidence to support its claims, but many herbs have since turned out to have uses much the same as those described in the 16th and 17th centuries. Lungwort does indeed help ease respiratory ailments, and pilewort ointment helps to constrict and ease swollen veins. Even viper's bugloss turns out to have some value in the treatment of snake bites. So despite the attitudes of modern science and medicine, perhaps we should learn to credit the ancient herbalists with more wisdom than we sometimes recognize.

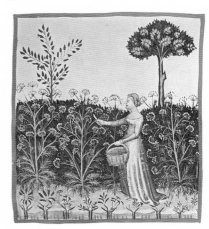

ABOVE *A young woman gathers the flowers of fennel from an herb garden.*

Herbal Practice

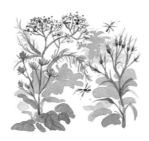

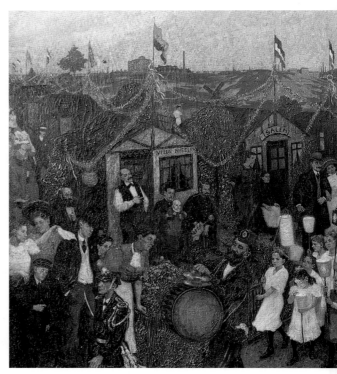

Herbs can be used in a variety of ways and for a variety of purposes; you may wish to celebrate a particular tradition, evoke an atmosphere, or simply flavor food. This section will give you all the basic preparation techniques you need in order to make the most of the herbs described in this book.

BELOW An herb candle can be made using your own selection of herbs.

Herbs can be used for many purposes such as healing, purification, and blessing rituals; in festive rites; and to help you to improve and enrich your lives, physically, emotionally, or spiritually. To maximize the positive effects of ritual herbs, you need to follow certain guidelines. Not only do many of these tips harness the most powerful essences of the herbs, but taking a spiritual approach to using them will help to focus your concentration, which is key to ensuring their effectiveness.

RIGHT Traditionally, lanterns are lit and herbs are burned at the Summer Solstice festival in June.

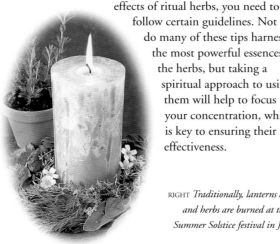

THE RITUAL USE OF HERBS

❧ Grow your own herbs if you are able to, or at least acquire them from friends who grow herbs themselves. (Buying fresh herbs at the supermarket has to be the very last resort.) Make sure they are grown naturally and organically, and as far as possible don't force the plants, but grow them naturally outdoors where the sun and the rain can warm and refresh them – and always use them in season.

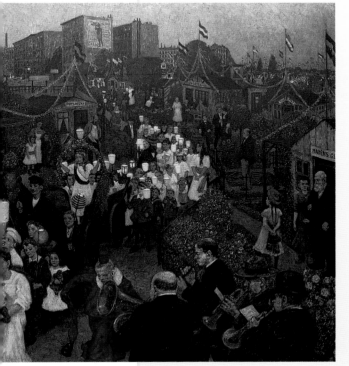

RIGHT Basil grown in pots will provide a constant supply of fresh leaves.

❧ Pick the herbs yourself, and do it in a happy and relaxed frame of mind. Pick them while the dew is still on them, when they are at their most potent. If you are not using the flowers, pick the herb before it has begun to bloom. Take a moment to enjoy the plant before you pick the parts you need.

❧ Treat the herbs with respect while you are preparing them for use; if you aren't going to prepare them immediately, put them in water in the meantime. While you are preparing the herbs for whatever purpose – drying, infusing, making into a wreath, or anything else – focus on the purpose of the herb and the end you hope to achieve. If any parts of the herb are left over after preparation, such as unused stalks or leaves, return these to the earth to go back into the soil. Don't just put them in the trash can.

❧ When you are ready to use the herbs, continue to treat them respectfully and focus again on your aim. Make sure you put as much effort into the other materials and equipment you use with them. Don't distill the oil from herbs and then place it in a chipped, dirty bottle – look for an elegant container. Find an attractive ribbon to tie around a posy, or choose an appropriate colored candle for a meditation ritual involving the use of herbs.

ABOVE Herbs make a beautiful addition to a garland.

BELOW A simple bundle of lavender tied with an attractive ribbon can brighten any room and bring a refreshing fragrance to it.

Growing Herbs in Tune with Nature's Rhythms

The moon regulates many aspects of life, the most obvious and well-documented being the tides. It has long been held that the most effective way to organize any activities in the garden, such as planting and harvesting, is to try to time them to coincide with the most beneficial phase of the moon's cycle.

For the first two quarters the moon is waxing, and for the third and fourth quarters it is waning. As a general guide, activities to promote growth, such as planting and fertilizing, should be done while the moon is waxing; pruning, harvesting, and those activities that reduce the herb should be done when the moon is on the wane.

However, there are some exceptions: harvesting herbs to be used immediately instead of preserved or stored, should be done during a waxing moon. Also, herbs that you are growing for their roots, such as horseradish or orris, should be planted during a waning moon.

BELOW *The moon is universally considered to have a powerful effect upon nature and her cycles.*

THE LUNAR CYCLE IS DIVIDED INTO FOUR SECTIONS

 THE FIRST QUARTER, from when the moon is new to when it is halfway to being full

 THE SECOND QUARTER, from when the moon is half full until the full moon

 THE THIRD QUARTER, from full moon to when it is halfway to being new

 THE FOURTH QUARTER, from when the moon is half way to being new until the new moon

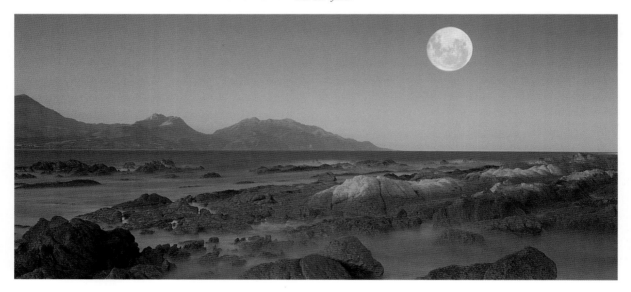

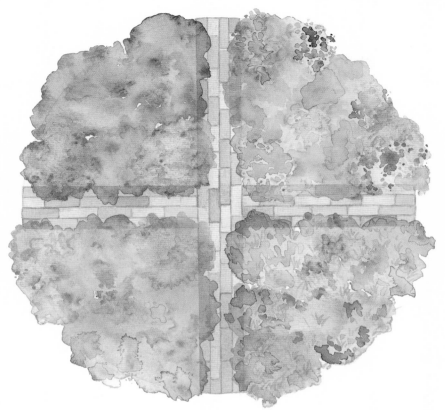

LEFT *The traditional herb garden tends to have geometric designs.*

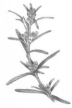

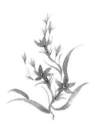

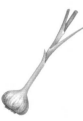

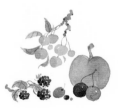

FIRST QUARTER

Plant any herbs that you grow for their leaves

Plant seeds

Prick out seedlings

Repot container grown herbs

SECOND QUARTER

Pick herbs for using immediately

Plant herbs that you grow for their flowers, fruits, or seeds

Plant all annual herbs

Fertilize with organic fertilizer as close to the full moon as possible

THIRD QUARTER

Plant herbs that you grow for the below-ground parts

Plant bulbous herbs

Cut and prune plants

Weed

Harvest herbs for storing and preserving

FOURTH QUARTER

Weed

Thin out plants

Companion Planting with Herbs

The principle behind companion planting is that certain plants will help to cultivate others if they are planted close by. This is usually effective because one plant controls pests that might otherwise attack the companion plant. This is a far more natural and, of course, organic approach to pest control than spraying pesticides or fungicides.

Some companion plants are effective because they attract pollinators, which then help to pollinate the neighboring plants. For example, borage, bergamot (also known as bee-balm), hyssop, summer savory, and thyme all attract bees in large numbers, and are therefore usefully planted among beans, tomatoes, and squash and their relatives, all of which need to be pollinated in order to produce crops.

Pollination is not the only reason to attract insects. Many insects produce larvae that feed on aphids, so you want to encourage them to lay their eggs on the plants that are susceptible to aphids. Hoverflies are very beneficial to the garden for this reason, and are attracted by umbelliferous herbs such as chervil, dill, or fennel.

Combating Pests

Many pests find the plants they are looking for by smell or by sight, and you can use herbs to confuse their senses and effectively hide the plant from them. Carrot aphids, for example, smell out its host plant. So if you interplant your carrots with a strongly aromatic herb, such as southernwood, you may well baffle the insects.

Other pests, such as cabbage-root fly, recognize the shape of the plants they are seeking outlined against the earth. Almost any kind of interplanting, particularly of a ground cover plant, will help to disguise the brassicas.

If you can't deter pests, another option is to plant an herb that acts as a decoy. Nasturtiums, for example, are often planted among beans because they are even more attractive to aphids, and therefore lure them away from the beans. Not only that, but they also make a beautiful plant combination to look at.

ABOVE *Planning a successful garden involves an understanding of the relationship between vegetables, flowers, and herbs.*

USEFUL HERBS FOR COMPANION PLANTING

HERB	COMPANION TO	FUNCTION
BASIL	tomatoes	repels insects
BORAGE	strawberries	increases yield
CAMOMILE	onions	increases yield
CHIVES	apple trees	prevents scab
FRENCH MARIGOLD	tomatoes	repels aphids
HYSSOP	grapes	increases yield
MINT	any plant	repels flies
NASTURTIUM	brassicas, beans, tomatoes	repels aphids
NETTLE	any plant	repels aphids
PENNYROYAL	any plant	repels ants
ROSEMARY	carrots	repels aphids
SAGE	any plant	repels many flying insects

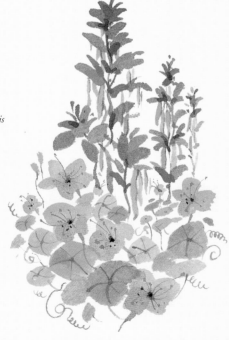

RIGHT *Beans rise up behind an abundance of nasturtiums in this companion planting.*

Medicinal Preparations from Herbs

If you choose to make your own herbal preparations, you will find that different ailments call for different types of remedy – infusions, compresses, oils, and so on. Whichever you need, you should harvest the herb in the morning if possible, and use it while it is still very fresh. If you are storing some or all of it instead of using it immediately, keep it in an airtight container or bottle; label and date it clearly and store it somewhere dark and cool.

BELOW You can make your own herbal creams by adding an essential oil of your choice to an unperfumed base cream such as lanolin.

PREPARATIONS YOU CAN MAKE AT HOME

COMPRESS: this enables you to apply a herb directly to the skin. Compresses can be hot or cold. A hot compress is made by heating a decoction or infusion (see below), soaking a cloth in it and holding it against the skin, or securing it with a bandage. It should be as hot as is bearable. If a cold compress is needed, simply let the hot compress cool down before using it.

CREAM: if you want to apply an herbal cream, simply add a few drops of the necessary essential oil to an unperfumed, plain cream such as lanolin or cocoa butter.

DECOCTION: using about 1oz. (30g) of the herb to 1 pint (500ml) of water, place the bruised herb in the water in a pan. Cover and bring to a boil. Remove the lid and simmer until the liquid has reduced to about a quarter of its original volume. Remove the pan from the heat, replace the lid, and leave it until it has cooled. A decoction will keep for around three days in the refrigerator. To use, strain the liquid.

ESSENTIAL OIL: these are simpler to buy than to make; a good selection is available from health food stores.

INFUSION: add the herb to boiling water and leave it to cool. Strain before using. Herbal teas are a type of infusion (see right).

POULTICE: this is similar to a compress, but you apply the herb itself, crushed and mixed with a little boiling water, directly to the skin in the same way as a compress.

TINCTURE: Add 8 oz. (225g) of fresh, chopped herb to 1 pint (500ml) of alcohol such as brandy. Put it in a warm place for two or three weeks, and shake it twice a day. Then strain it, and keep in an airtight bottle or jar in a dark place.

ABOVE To make a tincture, add fresh herbs to alcohol such as brandy and let it stand before straining and bottling it.

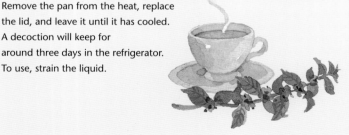

RIGHT Herbal tea is made by simply adding a few fresh herb leaves to boiling water.

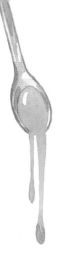

Tisanes to Improve your Health

A tisane is another name for a herbal tea; not an Indian or China tea with herbs added to it, but a tea made exclusively by infusing herbs in boiling water. Tisanes can be made from specific herbs for their healing properties, but any herbal tea has a health advantage over conventional tea simply because it contains no caffeine. When you make an herbal tea, you should avoid making it in the same teapot you use for Indian or China tea since the tannin deposits will inevitably mar the subtle flavor of the tisane.

Tisanes taste very different from conventional tea, and for many they are an acquired taste. They are drunk without milk but, if you prefer a sweet flavor, you can add honey. You can also add lemon juice or spices to the tisane if you wish (although it depends a little on the purpose of the tea – if you want a relaxant to help you sleep, lemon would counteract this).

Tisanes can be made using a single herb or a combination of herbs, depending on your taste and the purpose of the drink. Some people drink tisanes because they prefer them to conventional tea, in which case you can experiment until you find tea you like the taste of. If you want the tea for a specific medical purpose, however, you will need to choose an herb – or perhaps a combination of two or three herbs – that will give you the desired effect.

MAKING A TISANE

The method is very simple. Pour 1 pint (500ml) of boiling water over 2 teaspoons dried herbs, or about three times as much if you're using fresh herbs. Then leave it to steep for a few minutes before pouring it through a strainer. Once the tisane is in the cup, add any sweetener or spices you wish.

HERB COMBINATIONS TO ENJOY IN TISANES

REFRESHING MORNING TEA:
lemon balm, rose hip, and peppermint

SOOTHING TEA FOR SLEEP:
camomile, valerian, and hops

WARMING WINTER TEA:
camomile, cinnamon and apple (use sliced fresh apple)

BELOW *Another name for a dried herbal tea is a tisane.*

HEALTH GIVING PROPERTIES

HERB	FUNCTION
ANISEED	aids relaxation
BERGAMOT	eases coughs and colds
CARAWAY	eases digestion
CAMOMILE	aids relaxation
DANDELION	eases nausea
DILL	eases digestion
ELDERFLOWER	coughs, colds, and fever
FENNEL	eases digestion
LEMON BALM	eases coughs and colds

HERB	FUNCTION
MINT	tonic
NETTLE	tonic
RASPBERRY LEAF	eases menstrual cramps
SAGE	eases coughs and colds
SWEET CICELY	eases coughs and colds
TANSY	eases nausea
THYME	tonic
VERVAIN	reduces fever
YARROW	eases nausea

WARNING
Some herbs may be unsafe if taken during pregnancy. If you think you may be pregnant, check with a qualified doctor or herbal practitioner before drinking herbal teas.

Cooking with Herbs

One of the delights of cooking is using herbs, which can hugely improve the flavor of dishes and can give them a freshness and an individuality that is hard to achieve otherwise. Ideally, you should use fresh herbs in season, since this is when they are at their strongest and most flavorsome. If you are adding them to food for their health-giving properties as well as for their taste, they should certainly be fresh. However, some strongly flavored herbs can be preserved through the winter in oil or by freezing (see right). Commercially prepared dried herbs sold in supermarkets are not worth using, since they lack flavor.

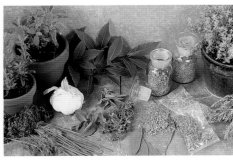

ABOVE *A variety of fresh and dried herbs should always be on hand in any kitchen.*

Generally speaking, herbs are best used singly so their individual, unique flavors can stand out. There are, however, some groups of herbs which work well together, in particular any combination of sage, marjoram, parsley, bay, and thyme is excellent for enhancing meaty dishes. Garlic and rosemary are both strong enough flavors to use in combination and still be able to taste each individually.

Suit the Herb to the Dish

Strong herbs will mask the flavor of delicate foods, so use milder herbs with light foods and strong herbs – often the oilier, evergreen ones – with more flavorful dishes. Cooking tends to kill the taste of herbs, so add mild herbs at the very end of the cooking process. Strong herbs, on the other hand, can be cooked for longer since they will retain enough of their flavor.

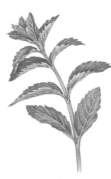

BELOW *Fresh mint has wonderful scented leaves.*

COMMON CULINARY HERBS AND SUGGESTED DISHES

HERB	USE FOR
BASIL	Mediterranean dishes, salads, tomatoes
CILANTRO	Spicy dishes, root vegetables
DILL	Fish, cream cheese
GARLIC	Almost anything, especially roasts
MARJORAM	Autumn stews, omelets
MINT	Lamb, new potatoes, peas, sweet dishes
PARSLEY	Sauces, eggs, fish
ROSEMARY	Red meat, root vegetables
SAGE	Strongly flavored dishes, winter stews
TARRAGON	Chicken, fish
THYME	All meats, winter stews

Smell is an important part of cooking, and cooking the herb with the rest of the dish certainly maximizes this. Think of the smell of lamb roasting with rosemary and garlic on a winter's day. If cooking gives a good smell but damages the flavor of the herb, add some at the start of the recipe for its smell, and a little more at the end to boost the flavor.

Preserving Herbs for the Winter

You may want to preserve herbs for cooking with through the winter, as an alternative to the seasonal herbs. Whatever method you use, you will need to start with very fresh herbs; don't pick them until the day you are ready to preserve them.

Drying Herbs

Only the strongest-tasting herbs are suitable for drying, such as bay or lovage. However, dried seeds of herbs such as fennel, dill, and caraway are worth collecting for cooking with. Simply hang the seed heads upside down over a piece of paper or cloth (preferably white, so you can see the seeds clearly), and when the seeds are ready they will fall out. Transfer them to airtight jars, where they will last all year.

ABOVE *The leaves of the bay tree can be harvested and dried, and bring added flavor to stew and sauces.*

To dry sprigs for cooking, clean the plants but avoid washing or wetting them if you possibly can. Hang the stems in small, loose bunches (so the air can circulate easily) in a warm dark place. They should be dry in about a week, but may take a little longer if the temperature is cooler.

Making Herb Oils

BELOW *Herbs can be chopped and frozen in ice cubes and enjoyed by those who want fresh herbs out of season.*

You can preserve many herbs in oil – obviously you will need to use them in recipes that can accommodate at least a teaspoon or two of oil. Fill a jar loosely with the fresh herb, and cover it with oil up to the top. Use a good-quality oil but avoid strong oils with subtly flavored herbs. Grapeseed or safflower oils are excellent, but you can use olive oil for garlic or Mediterranean herbs such as basil or oregano.

Place the jar in a sunny place. After two weeks, strain the mixture. If the flavor is not strong enough, repeat the process using the same oil with fresh herbs. When the herb oil is ready, transfer it to a clean bottle and label it. This should last you through the winter months.

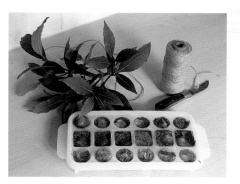

Freezing Herbs

Some recipes may be difficult to incorporate oil into, but can easily take a teaspoon of water. So another method of preserving is to put a teaspoon of chopped herbs into each compartment of an ice cube tray, top them up with water, and freeze them. When they're solid, transfer the frozen cubes to a bag, label them, and store them in the freezer. Simply add a cube of the herb you require to soups, stews, and sauces. This method preserves the flavor of leaf herbs far better than the traditional method of drying.

Beauty Treatments from Herbs

Many herbs have properties that are excellent for the skin, hair, eyes, and teeth. With creams and compresses, shampoos and essential oils, you can create a selection of herbal preparations to enhance and beautify yourself naturally. If you're making a cream, shampoo, or toner using herbs, the simplest method is to buy a pure product, that is free from fragrance, color and additives, and customize it. A plain lanolin cream, baby shampoo, or witch-hazel toner can be used as a base, and you can add the appropriate herb fresh, as an infusion or decoction, or as an essential oil.

EYES

To refresh the eyes or reduce puffiness, make two cold compresses and place over your closed eyes while you lie down for a few minutes.

FACE PACK

For a face pack, oatmeal and rosewater or elderflower water make an excellent base; simply mix to the right consistency.

HAIR RINSE

You can make a hair rinse simply by stirring a spoonful of cider or wine vinegar into a suitable, cooled herbal infusion, then pouring it over the hair after shampooing. Catch the rinse in a bowl held under your hair, and repeat several times.

TEETH

The teeth can be cleaned simply by rubbing a sage leaf or a cut strawberry over them.

HERBAL BATH

If you want to add herbs to the bath, simply put the fresh herb in a small cheesecloth drawstring bag, and hang it under the faucet as you run a hot bath.

RIGHT *Herbs and their functions are complex; there is not one part of the body that cannot benefit from the goodness of herbs.*

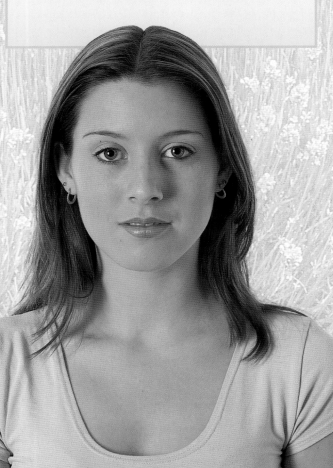

HERBS FOR BEAUTY

The following table gives you a general guide to which herbs can be used in which beauty treatments.

HERB	SKIN	HAIR	EYES	TEETH	BATH
CAMOMILE – *soothing*	✿	for dandruff	✿		✿
COMFREY – *healing*	✿	for dry hair			
DANDELION – *tonic*					✿
ELDERFLOWER – *tonic*	✿	for dry hair			
FENNEL – *cleansing*	✿		✿		✿
LAVENDER – *tonic*	✿	for greasy hair			✿
LEMON BALM – *tonic*		for greasy hair			✿
MARIGOLD – *healing*		for greasy hair	✿		✿
MINT – TONIC	✿	for greasy hair	✿	✿	✿
NETTLE – CLEANSING	for oily skin	for dry hair and dandruff			✿
ROSEMARY – *antiseptic, tonic, cleansing*	✿	for greasy hair			✿
SAGE – *cleansing, tonic*	✿	for dry hair		✿	✿
THYME – *antiseptic, cleansing*	✿	for dandruff			✿
VALERIAN – *soothing*					✿
YARROW – *healing, cleansing*	✿	for greasy hair			✿

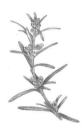

ABOVE Rosemary infusion can be used as a disinfectant.

BELOW Herbs have featured in kitchens for many centuries, and not just to flavor the food.

Herbs for Cleansing and Strewing

In the days when disease was rife and chemical disinfectant cleaner was not being manufactured, people used herbs to cleanse and refresh their homes. Naturally antiseptic herbs were used in infusions for washing floors and kitchen tables, and herbs were strewn on the floor to bring fresh, clean smells indoors. Other herbs were placed in folded linen or clothes, or put in bowls. In a sense, these were early – and natural – air fresheners.

Antiseptic Herbs

Many herbs have natural antiseptic qualities, which can be harnessed. Infusions of these herbs used for cleaning, or bowls and vases of fresh herbs, help to bring freshness to the house. Antiseptic herbs include fennel, garlic, golden-rod, hyssop, marjoram, mint, rosemary, sage, southern wood, and thyme. An infusion of rosemary makes a particularly good disinfectant, and you can add it to unscented dishwashing detergent if you want to use it to remove grease.

HERBAL PEST CONTROL

Some herbs act as excellent insect repellents and have traditionally been used to discourage all sorts of household pests:

FLEAS: fleabane, burned slowly to fumigate the infested area

ANTS: sprigs of rue or tansy

MICE: sprigs of mint or tansy

FLIES: lavender, mint, rue, or southernwood hung in a bunch or placed in a bowl

FLOUR WEEVILS: bay leaves

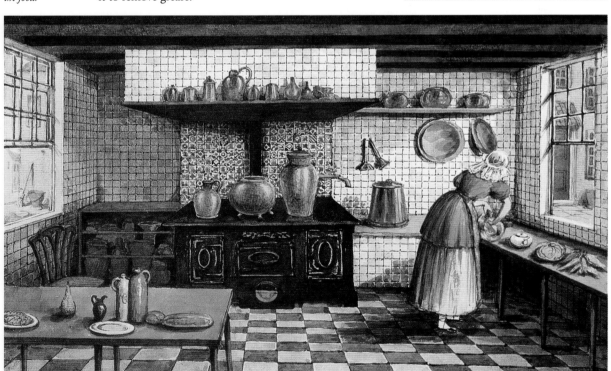

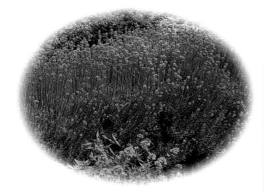

RIGHT *Lavender is a popular herb because it promotes relaxation. It grows outdoors even in colder climates.*

Strewing Herbs

Strewing herbs were used on the floor and were generally absorbent as well as antiseptic and sweet smelling. Treading on them helped to release their scent. Nowadays, vases of fresh herbs, or bunches of them hung up to dry, may be more practical than herbs strewn on the floor. Sweet rushes, lavender, santolina, southernwood, and tansy were among the most popular strewing herbs, and in the winter, evergreens such as juniper were used.

Lavender is perhaps the most popular of all herbs for refreshing the house, partly because it retains its scent well even after it has been dried. Lavender not only smells sweet, it also promotes relaxation; and placed inside a pillow it encourages sleep. Lavender bags – little sachets containing dried lavender flowers – were used among clothes and other fabrics to keep them fresh and to keep moths and other insects away. The flowers scattered on books prevent them from smelling musty, and bunches of dried lavender tied with ribbon can be hung around the house.

LAVENDER SACHET

Cut out squares or heart shapes of fine cotton or organza. Place two pieces back to back and machine-stitch three sides together, leaving a small seam. Turn right side out, then add dried lavender to fill the sachets loosely. Add a drop of lavender oil to each, then sew up the open sides.

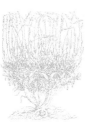

ABOVE *Lavender is a favorite for homemade* potpourri.

LAVENDER BAGS

You will need:

ORGANZA, FINE NET, OR GAUZE

THIN RIBBON

DRIED LAVENDER FLOWERS

LAVENDER OIL

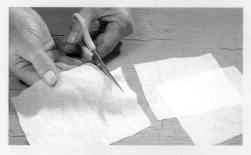

1 Cut squares, about 5in. (12cm) in size, from the fabric.

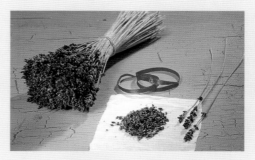

2 Place a small mound of dried lavender flowers in the middle of each square. Drop a little lavender essential oil onto the dried herb to enhance its scent.

3 Gather up the material around the lavender, twist to secure it, then tie up with the ribbon.

Harnessing the Power of Herbal Scents and Smells

Smell is a very powerful sense, and the scent of many herbs can be used to influence the mood beneficially. Scientific research has shown that herbal scents are very effective for treating negative emotional states such as anxiety and depression; nerves in the olfactory system are linked directly to the parts of the brain which control emotion. No wonder a fleeting smell can bring back emotive memories.

There are several ways in which scents can be derived from herbs and released into a room. The most obvious is simply to place a bunch of fresh, scented herbs in a vase of water. You can also heat essential oils over a candle flame to release the smell, put a few drops in the bath water, or add them to massage oils and apply the oil directly to the skin.

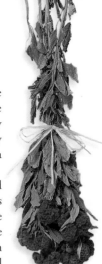

ABOVE *A simple bunch of dried scented roses can be hung around your house to give out a rich, enduring perfume.*

Potpourri

Potpourris – bowls of dried, scented herbs – have been used for thousands of years, and they are still made just as they always were. One of the most important ingredients is orris root powder, made from the root of the Florentine iris (*Iris florentina*). This has a gentle violet scent, and acts as a fixative, helping the other herbs to hold their scent. You can buy powdered orris root from a good herbal supplier.

ABOVE *The scent of herbs is easily released into a room; simply add a few drops of essential oil to a burning candle and let its aroma surround you.*

PREPARING YOUR OWN POTPOURRI

1 First dry each herbal ingredient separately.

2 Once dried, put about a 1 in. (2.5cm) layer of the herbs in a jar, then cover it with a layer of salt and orris root powder – about ½ teaspoon of each.

3 Continue to fill the jar in these layers until you have used up all the dried herbs.

4 Cover the jar with an airtight lid, then store it in a dark place for two or three weeks.

To use the potpourri, simply put a quantity of the dried herbs (with the salt and orris powder) into a bowl. Add just a few drops of one, or perhaps two, essential oils of your choice, and stir it all together. If you like, you can add spices such as cinnamon and cloves, or even dried citrus peel.

SPICY POTPOURRI

LAVENDER OIL

ROSEMARY LEAVES

BAY LEAVES (CRUSHED)

CARDAMOM SEEDS (CRUSHED)

CINNAMON STICKS (BRUISED)

CLOVES

ALLSPICE BERRIES (CRUSHED)

LEMON PEEL

RELAXING POTPOURRI

LAVENDER FLOWERS

ROSE PETALS

DIANTHUS PETALS

SOUTHERNWOOD LEAVES

VANILLA PODS (BRUISED)

HOPS

REFRESHING POTPOURRI

GINGER OIL

PEPPERMINT LEAVES

SPEARMINT LEAVES

LEMON VERBENA LEAVES

LEMON BALM LEAVES

THYME LEAVES

ORANGE PEEL

BERGAMOT OIL

THYME OIL

Making Posies, Wreaths, and Garlands

Flowers and herbs have been used to make attractive displays for thousands of years in cultures across the world. But their purpose is not always purely decorative. Often, flowers and herbs are cut and included in posies, wreaths, or garlands because of their sacred properties or medicinal qualities, and this is the origin of arrangements such as garlands, wreaths, and posies.

Garlands and wreaths are usually made for ritual purposes. Their circular shape – without beginning or end – symbolizes eternity and the constant cycle of the seasons, or of life and death. If you think about it, this ritual shape could have been traditionally sculpted out of almost anything, but flowers have always been chosen because they, too, represent natural cycles. Wreaths are used in funeral rites to encourage the smooth transition from this world to the next of the person who has passed away; garlands create a circular link in a chain that links people together, so they are a symbol of friendship.

Including herbs in wreaths and garlands – sometimes making them exclusively of herbs – gives the maker an opportunity to weave in symbols of their choice. A funeral wreath, for example, can include herbs associated with death such as thyme, anemone, and ivy, and others with pertinent symbolic meanings such as morning glory leaves for rebirth, rosemary for remembrance, and lilies for peace.

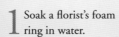

LEFT *The herb thyme is associated with death and can be included in funeral wreaths.*

A FRESH CHRISTMAS WREATH

You will need:

1 FLORIST'S FOAM RING	RED OR BLUE RIBBON, WITH GOLD TRIM
SCISSORS	
FLORIST'S WIRE	SPRIGS OF HOLLY, VARIEGATED IVY, ROSEMARY (FLOWERING IF POSSIBLE), OR ROSE HIPS

1 Soak a florist's foam ring in water.

2 Insert the stems of sprigs of holly and variegated ivy into the foam, until it is well covered.

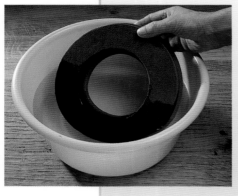

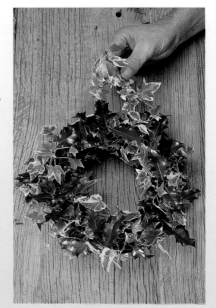

Posies

A posy is a carefully selected collection of herbs or flowers bound together in a compact bunch around a central flower or stem. Traditionally, posies were often made as a kind of portable medicine; the sweet smell was thought to ward off disease and illness. Many people carried them during outbreaks of the plague to protect them against the noxious fumes of disease. These posies consisted of such herbs as lavender, rosemary, lemon balm, pinks, and sage, tied around a central bloom, such as a rose.

Posies are still exchanged today, although for less sinister reasons – to represent protection or purification. They should be gathered at a suitably propitious time and hung upside down to dry. For example, a posy for blessing the household might be picked at midsummer and centered around a sprig of St. John's wort, the herb of the sun. The posy will then bestow its goodwill on the household for a year, at the end of which it should be replaced with a fresh posy.

If a posy is needed for ritual purification, it should be collected a few months in advance and taken down when needed. It should then be placed in a pan, lit, and carried all around the house. Make sure you leave out no rooms, however small, or they will not be purified.

ABOVE *Posies were carried by people in the belief that they would protect against the plague and other contagious diseases in the midst of urban squalor.*

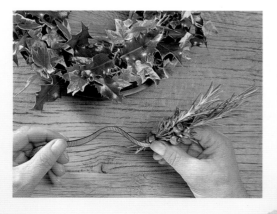

4 Spray with water occasionally and replace only wilted leaves.

3 Tie together sprigs of rosemary or rose hips with florist's wire and finish with red or blue and gold ribbon. Insert into the foam.

Aries

MARCH 21 – APRIL 20

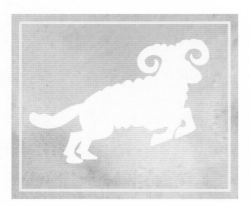

"HE IS THE CAPTAIN, THE LEADER, PIONEER AMONG MEN; GOING OUT IN SYMPATHY TO A NEW THOUGHT, RAPIDLY ASSIMILATING FRESH IDEAS, ALWAYS IN THE VAN OF PROGRESS IN WHATEVER KIND OF WORK — INTELLECTUAL, ARTISTIC OR PRACTICAL — HE MAY TAKE UP."

ISABELLE M. PAGAN *FROM PIONEER TO POET*

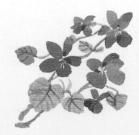

VIOLET, THE LOVE HERB

Masculine, aggressive, decisive, and energetic, the planet Mars rules the sign of Aries. The three key herbs of Aries are garlic, rosemary, and cowslip. In the following pages you will discover how these herbs can enhance your life. First, though, it is interesting to look at the herbs in season at this time of year, and the role they play in the traditional festivals and rituals that fall under the Aries cycle.

Seasonal Rites

The vernal equinox, on March 21st or 22nd, marks the sun's entry into the sign of Aries. This is the time of year when the hours of daylight and darkness are equal in length. From this time on, the days become longer, so the festival of the equinox marks the start of the astrological year, and the flowering of the spring.

The growth of the first flowers, after the winter dearth, brings a feeling of joy and rejuvenation. The most important flowers used in spring festival rituals are the abundance of yellow flowers that grow at this time of the year; their color

The flush of spring is the time when the mind turns to love, and one of the most potent love herbs is the violet, which flowers at this time of year. The violet has heart-shaped leaves, and its scent encourages thought or contemplation. Give a posy of them to your loved one before he or she leaves on a journey; it will encourage them to remember you while they are gone.

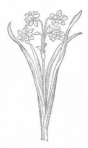

ABOVE *The yellow jonquil celebrates the flowering of spring.*

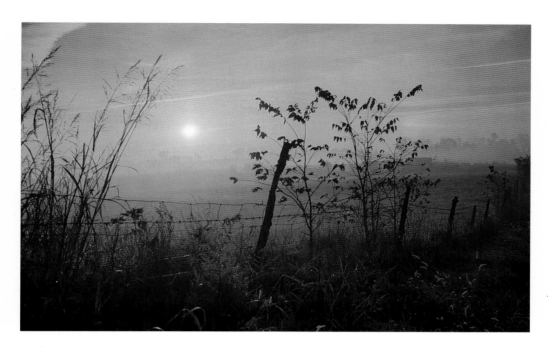

LEFT *Taking place just before sunrise, the spring equinox rites traditionally celebrate the start of longer daylight hours.*

represents the sun, which is coming into its strength. Primroses, cowslips, daffodils, and jonquils all celebrate the new year, and are used to decorate the place where the spring ritual is held.

The purpose of the spring equinox rites was to say goodbye to the darkness and welcome the return of longer daylight hours. The ritual took place just before sunrise; people used to gather and meditate upon the winter which had just passed. A moment or two before dawn, they wished darkness farewell and greeted the sun with joyous shouts and dancing.

ARIES COMPLAINTS

People born under Aries are natural leaders. In medical astrology this sign governs the head and is associated with illnesses such as headaches, sinus problems, eye conditions, ear infections, and conditions relating to the hair, from dandruff to baldness. Aries people are particularly prone to these kind of complaints, and even to accidents involving the head – they often bump into things. It does not necessarily follow that the Aries herbs are the most appropriate herbs to cure these problems – for the most useful herbs to help Aries complaints, *see pages 124–127.*

RIGHT *Those born under Aries are likely to suffer from complaints that affect the scalp and hair.*

Garlic

Long recognized for its medicinal and therapeutic qualities, garlic has been cultivated in the East for at least 4,000 years and was grown by the ancient Egyptians. Indeed, the Romans issued garlic cloves to their soldiers on a daily basis, to keep up their strength.

Healing with Garlic

Garlic has a wide range of active ingredients that give it many important medicinal qualities. In addition to the active constituents of its oil, it also contains vitamins A, B_1, B_2, and C.

Garlic is used to reduce blood pressure, help digestion, ease coughs and colds, and generally help build up the body's own ability to fight illness. It also has antiseptic properties and was used for economy in both world wars as a poultice applied to wounds to help prevent gangrene and blood poisoning. The old superstition that garlic can destroy the magnetic power of the lodestone is cited by Pliny and Plutarch.

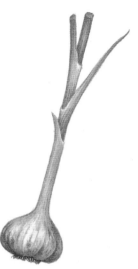

ABOVE *Garlic is a bulbous-rooted herb originally most popular in Europe and now used worldwide.*

ABOVE *Wild garlic has small, sweet-tasting cloves.*

SAFE FROM VAMPIRES

So many properties were attributed to garlic that it was used as a charm against the evil eye. The Scots carried it for protection on All Hallows Eve, or Samhain – the night when the dead are said to walk. It was this custom that led to its adoption as a protection against vampires. The superstition is Slavonic, but was popularized by horror stories like Bram Stoker's *Dracula*.

RIGHT *The classic vampire scenario shows the monster preying on beautiful young women for their blood.*

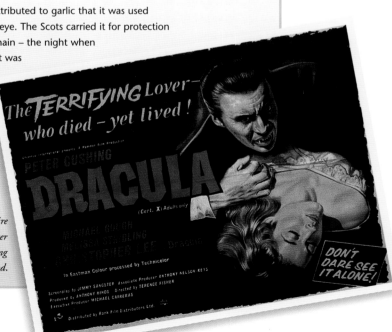

The TERRIFYING Lover – who died – yet lived !

PETER CUSHING

DRACULA

(Cert. X) Adults only

MICHAEL GOUGH
MELISSA STRIBLING
AND CHRISTOPHER LEE as Dracula

In Eastman Colour processed by Technicolor

Screenplay by JIMMY SANGSTER Associate Producer ANTHONY NELSON KEYS
Produced by ANTHONY HINDS Directed by TERENCE FISHER
Executive Producer MICHAEL CARRERAS

Distributed by Rank Film Distributors Ltd.

DON'T DARE SEE IT ALONE!

GARLIC AS A SEASONING

Garlic is a popular seasoning especially to accompany meat. Traditionally, it has been used in Mediterranean cooking, although nowadays it is used just as often in British and American kitchens.

Whole roast garlic cloves lose much of their pungency and acquire a sweet, rich flavor which complements most baked food, from meat to fish and vegetables.

Try harvesting wild garlic, which has much smaller cloves but tastes sweeter.

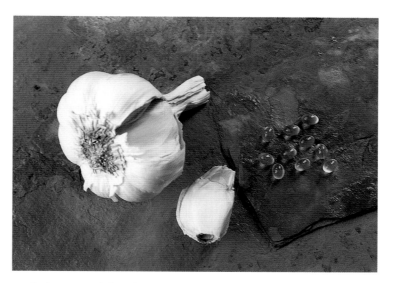

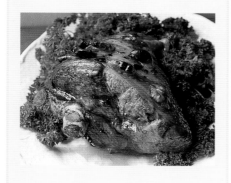

ABOVE *Whole cloves, stripped of their white skin, can be placed in cuts in a roast of lamb. Alternatively, add crushed garlic to oil and baste the meat.*

Garlic is one of those herbs that has a well-deserved reputation as a cure-all. It has proved successful in treating dysentery and diarrhea, diphtheria, TB, whooping cough, typhoid, hepatitis, and even worms. It lowers blood sugar levels, which makes it useful in the treatment of diabetes. People have long claimed that it helps in the treatment of cancer, and scientific research is now showing that there may be some basis for this folk belief.

Many people take daily garlic supplements to strengthen their immune system and protect against heart disease.

ABOVE *Garlic is known as a "cure-all," and regular doses keep many illnesses at bay.*

SWEET BREATH

Some people love the taste of garlic but feel uncomfortable about the smell that lingers on the breath. To avoid this problem, eat a sprig or two of raw parsley, which neutralizes the smell.

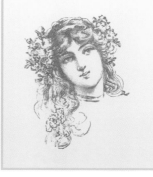

Cooking with Garlic

Garlic is used widely to add flavor to many dishes; this is the best way to reap the benefits of its medicinal uses, too. It can be used raw, although this makes its taste much stronger. Cooking tones down the flavor without damaging its health-giving properties. Add garlic, sliced or crushed, to stews, soups, sauces, and dressings.

Cook whole peeled cloves with baked vegetables and meats. These can be served with the meal. Slip a few cloves into cuts in the skin of a cut of lamb before you cook it, or inside a chicken before putting it in the oven. You can even roast whole heads of garlic as a vegetable in their own right.

Rosemary

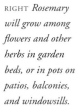

A popular, aromatic garden herb, rosemary has pointed, bright green leaves and attractive blue flowers. It is a very useful herb since it has many properties, both medicinal and culinary, and because it is an evergreen, it is available fresh all year round. It was first used by the ancient Egyptians, and its medicinal and culinary properties have been exploited ever since.

Future and Friendship

Rosemary is an important ritual herb and, like many other herbs that are regarded as sacred, it has folk uses for divination. For example, it is said that if a young woman places a flat plate or dish of flour underneath a rosemary bush on Midsummer's Eve, she will find her future husband's initials etched in it the next morning.

Rosemary represents friendship in popular folklore, and it is said that if you grow a rosemary bush in your yard, you are protected from evil, since only friends can come near you. You will never be short of friends if your yard contains rosemary. On the other hand, you may not be able to grow it at all, since another popular belief about rosemary is that it only flourishes in the yard of a house where the woman is the dominant figure in the household.

ABOVE *The spiky leaves of the Rosemary bush are highly aromatic.*

RIGHT *Rosemary will grow among flowers and other herbs in garden beds, or in pots on patios, balconies, and windowsills.*

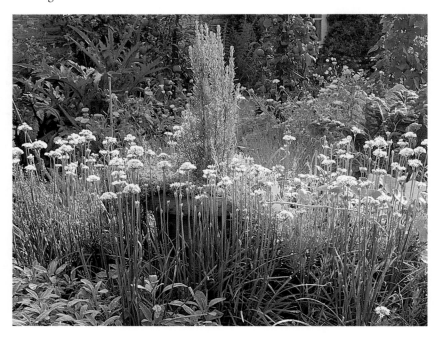

Healing with Rosemary

A useful healing herb, rosemary is particularly valuable in the treatment of headaches. It is the leaf that is used medicinally; alternatively, the oil extracted from the leaf can be used for direct application.

Rosemary oil applied to the head has the ability to ease a headache because it stimulates the blood supply to the area.

The oil's ability to stimulate the blood can also be used to help poor circulation. It can be added to a morning bath as a revitalizer. In addition, the stimulant effects of rosemary can aid sluggish digestion, by helping to pep up the liver and gall bladder, and thus easing flatulence.

Rosemary is generally taken as a tea, or simply added to food during cooking. The essential oil, like all essential oils, should only be used externally.

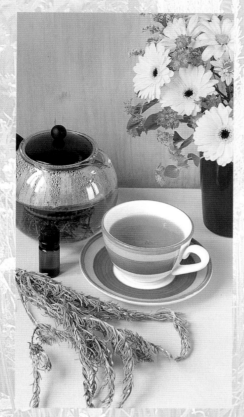

RIGHT *Rosemary is commonly taken as an herbal tea or added to food during cooking.*

WARNING
Rosemary should be used with care, if at all, during pregnancy.

ROSEMARY AS AN AROMATIC HERB

Rosemary plays a key role as an incense (its old French name was *incensier*) during the festival rites for welcoming in spring. The rosemary sprigs are gathered, tied together in bunches, and dried. These bundles are then lit, and the flames are extinguished, so that the bundle smolders, releasing a strong, cleansing scent.

The significance of rosemary incense is to cleanse the fresh, new year of the darkness of the preceding winter. But it has a dual role, because rosemary is also the herb of remembrance. Even as the new year is cleansed, the rosemary guarantees that the old year and the darkness of winter are not forgotten; but are merely consigned to the past as life moves on. Rosemary acts in the ritual as a reminder that we should learn from the past but not dwell on it – taking the opportunity to look afresh at life.

Cooking with Rosemary

Rosemary is an invaluable culinary herb, not least because it is an evergreen and can therefore be used throughout the winter when many other herbs are below ground. Its distinctive aroma is particularly strong during cooking, and it is enough to make your mouth water before you even taste it. Its flavor is quite powerful, so it is best combined with moderate to strong-flavored meat. The herb goes particularly well with lamb, or you can put a few sprigs inside a chicken, perhaps with a couple of halved lemons, before baking it.

Rosemary need not be restricted to meat dishes alone; it also tastes delicious with root vegetables. Try baking sprigs of rosemary with potatoes, carrots, turnips, sweet potatoes, or parsnips. Add the herb to winter stews and soups for extra aroma.

COOKING TIP

Some people enjoy the flavor of rosemary but find the leaves a little tough to eat. Either chop them very finely, or strain them out of soup and gravy before serving. For stews, tie together a small bundle of rosemary sprigs before adding them to the pot, so that you can remove the herb easily before serving.

ROSEMARY AND GARLIC ROAST POTATOES

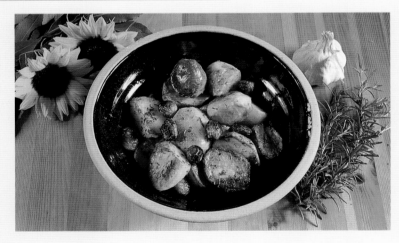

Serves 4

6 MEDIUM-SIZED POTATOES

1 HEAD OF GARLIC

3–4 SPRIGS OF ROSEMARY

5OZ. (150ML) SUNFLOWER OR LIGHT OLIVE OIL (OR THE FAT FROM THE ROAST)

1 Preheat the oven to 200°C/400°F.

2 Peel the potatoes and cut each one into about eight pieces. Peel the garlic cloves.

3 Finely chop the sprigs of rosemary.

4 Boil the potatoes and garlic together until they are slightly cooked.

5 Strain the potatoes and garlic, and leave to dry for a few minutes.

6 Put the potatoes and garlic in a baking dish; coat them with oil. Sprinkle chopped rosemary over them.

7 Bake in the oven for about 1 hour, turning occasionally, until they are golden and crisp.

Cowslip

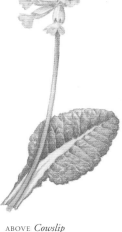

Found growing wild in fields and pastures, cowslips have yellow flowers that are delicately fragrant. The flowers come in a variety of slightly different shapes, some with distorted calyces. This has given rise to many of their common names, "St. Peter's keys," "Our Lady's keys," and "culverkeys" to mention a few. The keylike shape of the cowslip flowers may be the reason why the plant was traditionally thought to have the power to split open rocks that contained hidden treasure; or perhaps it was the golden color of the flowers that gave rise to the belief.

CHANGING FLOWER

According to custom, if you plant a cowslip upside-down, it will come up with a red flower – unless you plant it on Good Friday, in which case it will turn into a primrose You can also make your cowslips turn red – should you want to – by feeding them on bullocks' blood.

Healing with Cowslip

Cowslip flowers have sedative properties and can be made into a tea to help cure insomnia; cowslip wine has a similar soporific effect. A tea made from the flowers can also help ease inflammatory conditions that affect the throat and lungs, such as bronchitis. If it is made into a syrup, it also helps to soothe a cough.

Cooking with Cowslip

Cowslip is not widely used as a culinary herb. However, it is edible and the leaves can be used in salad or stuffing. The yellow flowers are also edible and can be crystallized, or used fresh as an edible decoration, bringing color to your chosen dish.

ABOVE *Cowslip grows wild in meadows and along river banks.*

RIGHT *Cowslip makes a pretty addition to any spring flower bed.*

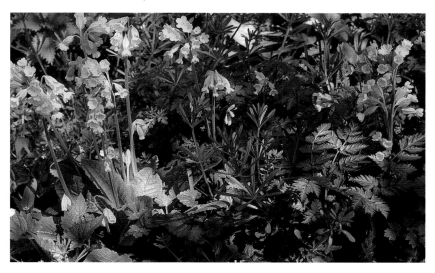

Taurus

APRIL 21 - MAY 21

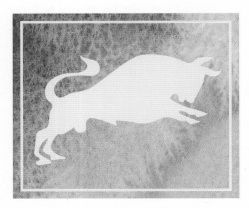

"The chief characteristic of the highly developed Taurean is his stability of character and of purpose. He is the steadfast mind, unshaken in adversity, and his the power of quiet persistence in the face of difficulties."

Isabelle M. Pagan *From Pioneer to Poet*

The word Taurus derives from the Latin for bull. This sign is ruled by the planet Venus, and the chief Taurus herbs are mint, lovage, and thyme. Before exploring the qualities of these herbs, it is interesting to know a little about the seasonal herbs within Taurus, and their role in the festivals and rituals celebrated at this time.

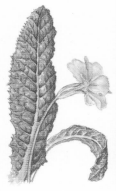

ABOVE *The delicate yellow of the primrose signifies the beginning of new life celebrated on May Day.*

Seasonal Rites

One of the year's most famous festivals, Beltane, falls within the sign of Taurus. Beltane falls on April 30th and celebrates the beginning of summer. Traditionally, bonfires were lit to honor the sun, and the festival would continue all night and into the next day. The Beltane fires were made from nine different types of wood, kindled by rubbing oak twigs together.

One of the most potent talismans for protecting against witches and evil spirits is the rowan, and a small stick can be kept in a pocket or purse all year round. These rowan branches were traditionally carried around the Beltane fire three times, pointed toward it, to strengthen their protective powers.

The day following Beltane is May Day, when the summer truly begins. The May Day festival celebrates the fertility and fecundity of this time of year, and this is symbolized with flowers. Green and yellow are the colors of summer and fresh life, and the herbs most associated with this festival are primroses and marsh marigolds (one of the local names for marsh marigold is "herb of Beltane").

ABOVE *Spring flowers: cow parsley, bluebell, cowslip, and dog rose.*

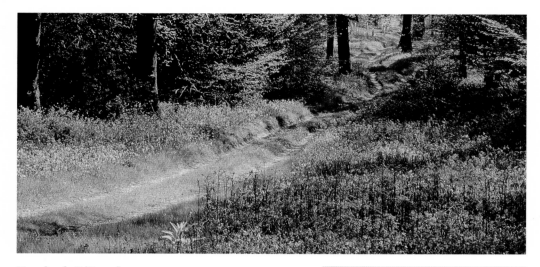

RIGHT *The astrological sign of Taurus occurs in late spring, when bluebells fill hedges and woodlands with a burst of color.*

Herbal Rituals

One of the village traditions associated with this festival was to carry flowers and herbs from house to house to keep away evil spirits and to bring good luck. May garlands were made from fresh flowers, such as cow parsley, bluebells, cowslips, primroses (if they were still flowering), and apple blossom, and carried from door to door on May Day to bless the houses and their occupants.

Another similar ritual involved collecting marsh marigolds on Beltane and placing one through each front door in the evening, to be found on May morning. It is unlucky to bring marsh marigolds into the house before May, but it is a lucky flower to keep on the table or windowsill through the early summer. Primroses were often used to protect cattle, and primroses inside the cowshed would prevent evil spirits from stealing the milk from the cows, as would a carpet of primroses and marsh marigolds strewn across the threshold.

Marsh marigolds can be hard to come by, especially if you don't live in the country, but if you want to practice your own Beltane rituals, you can use buttercups. Buttercups have always been associated with fertility, particularly in cattle. Taurus, of course, is the sign of the bull, and the beginning of May marks the time when cattle come into full milk.

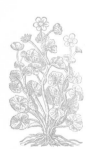

ABOVE *During Beltane rituals, Marsh Marigolds can be replaced by buttercups, which are also associated with fertility.*

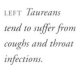

TAURUS COMPLAINTS

Influenced by the planet Venus, Taurus governs the neck and throat, and therefore illnesses such as sore throats, tonsillitis, laryngitis, and coughs. Taureans are not only prone to these kinds of illnesses, but also to overeating and therefore obesity – a tendency to guard against. It does not necessarily follow that the Taurus herbs are the best type for dealing with the problems that come under this sign – for the most useful herbs in treating Taurus complaints, see pages 124-127.

LEFT *Taureans tend to suffer from coughs and throat infections.*

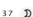

Mint

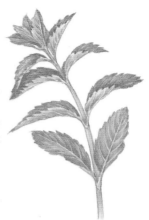

There are numerous species of mint, which are native to Europe and North America. Several originally came from the south of Europe, but were widely distributed by the Romans. Since different species of mint cross-fertilize easily, it is hard to be specific about the number of varieties that exist; but the most commonly used types are applemint, spearmint, and peppermint. If you grow several mints together, you will find they all inter-breed, unless you prevent them from flowering by removing the flowering tops before the buds open.

Healing with Mint

Almost all of mint's medicinal uses involve its ability to freshen and clear the air, either in the surrounding atmosphere or within the body. Spearmint and peppermint are the best mints to use medicinally, since their effects are strongest. Mint has many uses for colds, flu, sinus complaints, and other illnesses that cause congestion.

You can sprinkle drops of the essential oil on a handkerchief, or add it to a bowl of steaming water, and inhale to clear the sinuses and airways. An infusion, drunk as a tea, will help with colds and flu, and can also ease stomach ailments such as hiccups and flatulence.

BELOW *The common housefly is repelled by leaves of fresh mint.*

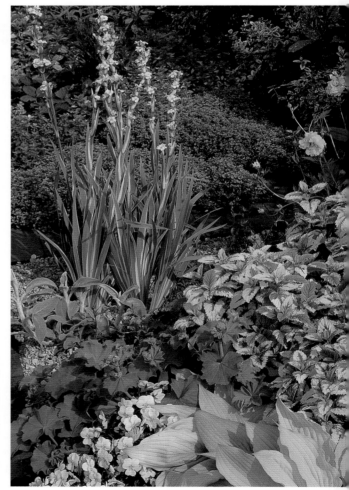

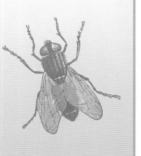

INSECT REPELLENT

Mint was traditionally used as an insect repellent, laid among clothing or bedding, or placed in the larder to repel ants.

Its scent is pungent and tends to fill rooms, so mint also helps to drive away flies. Keep a vase of mint sprigs on the kitchen windowsill.

Mint was traditionally believed to cure hay fever: some placed in your pillow and a sprig carried during the day freshens the air and brings about the cure.

Mint can also be pounded with oil and strained, and the resulting mint oil used as a rub on the face and temples to ease headaches, and on any part of the body to relieve muscular aches and pains.

Cooking with Mint

Mint adds a refreshing tang to many dishes, and is a very popular flavoring for sweet and non–sweet dishes. It is famously served as a sauce or jelly with roast lamb. The fresh leaves are traditionally cooked with new potatoes or peas to add flavor; mint has a strong enough flavor to cook with the vegetables without losing its potency – two or three sprigs are plenty.

There are numerous different mints, each with a slightly different flavor – ginger mint, orange mint, apple mint, eau de Cologne mint and so on – and you can experiment with different flavors. Spearmint is usually regarded as the best all-purpose culinary mint if you're only going to grow one variety.

Mixed with yogurt and finely chopped cucumber, it makes a light accompaniment to spicy foods such as curry or spicy meatballs. When it comes to sweet dishes, mint is most popularly paired with chocolate; fresh chopped mint can be added to a chocolate mousse, or crystallized mint sprigs can be used to decorate chocolate cakes. You can even make your own mint chocolates. Because of its cooling qualities, mint is also a popular flavoring to add to cold desserts such as sorbet and home-made ice cream.

BELOW *Mint is an especially enjoyable accompaniment to chocolate mousse.*

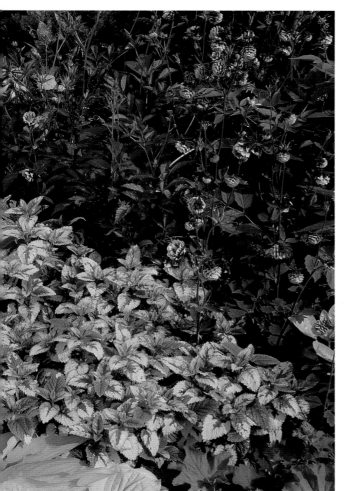

LEFT *Variegated mint dominates this herb border alongside hostas and violas.*

Lovage

Lovage has highly aromatic leaves with a powerful flavor. It is native to southern Europe, but was introduced to the rest of Europe and other continents centuries ago. Lovage was traditionally placed in the shoes of weary travelers to revive them, although it may be that the strong smell was more beneficial to others, since it would have masked any natural smell emanating from well-traveled shoes!

ABOVE *Lovage has culinary as well as medicinal qualities.*

LOVE SPELLS

Not surprisingly, given its name, lovage was most popular in folk tradition as an aphrodisiac, and was used to make love charms and potions. It was often made into a cordial, combined with tansy and yarrow, or the leaves were used in soups and stews, and served to the object of one's affections.

Healing with Lovage

Lovage can be taken as an infusion to treat a number of complaints. The leaves, seeds, or roots can be used; all possess the same properties.

Lovage is useful for settling the stomach and for easing the digestion and reducing flatulence. It is also said to be helpful in controlling migraines and rheumatism. Applied as a poultice or compress, lovage can help to ease mild dermatitis and so on.

WARNING
Lovage should be avoided during pregnancy.

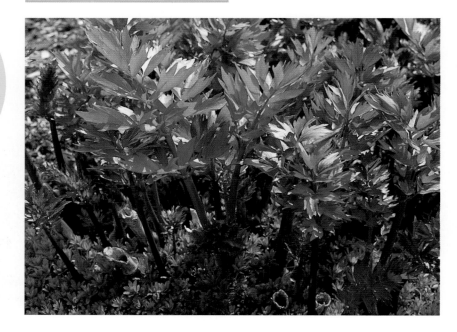

RIGHT *Lovage, growing here in abundance, has traditionally been served in food to win the heart of another.*

Cooking with Lovage

Lovage tastes a little like celery; the leaves, stems, roots, and seeds are all edible. The seeds can be sprinkled in salads or on home-baked bread, or used in rice dishes. The leaves, stems, and root can be used in soups and stews, or raw in salads; the flavor goes particularly well with cheese dishes. If you are not used to cooking with lovage, be warned: the flavor is very strong.

LOVAGE AND CELERY SOUP

Serves 4

6 TBL. (75G) BUTTER

1 BUNCH FRESH LOVAGE LEAVES AND STEMS, ROUGHLY CHOPPED

4 STICKS CELERY, ROUGHLY CHOPPED

1 HANDFUL PARSLEY, ROUGHLY CHOPPED

1 CLOVE GARLIC, FINELY CHOPPED

4 SLICES (50G) BROWN BREAD (NO CRUSTS)

3 PT. (1.5L) VEGETABLE BROTH (BOILING)

¾ PT (150ML) HEAVY CREAM

PINCH OF GRATED NUTMEG

SALT AND PEPPER TO TASTE

1 Melt butter in a saucepan.

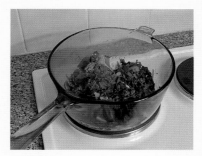

2 Gently cook the celery, parsley, and garlic in the butter for 3 or 4 minutes, without browning.

3 Add the lovage, nutmeg, salt, and pepper and cook for a further 2–3 minutes.

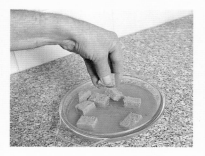

4 Soak the bread in a little broth for a couple of minutes. Squeeze out the bread and add it to the other ingredients in the pan.

5 Add the boiling broth slowly to the pan, stirring continuously. Then simmer for 10 minutes.

6 Liquidize the soup.

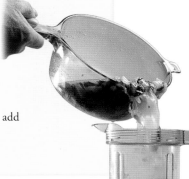

7 Reheat and, just before serving, remove from the heat and add the cream.

Thyme

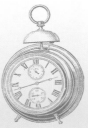

This well-known herb, native to Europe and northwestern Asia, has been cultivated for its culinary and medicinal uses since ancient times. Its name comes from the Greek meaning "courage," and it is traditionally worn – especially by soldiers – to impart bravery. Roman soldiers wore it, as did Crusaders in the Middle Ages.

Healing with Thyme

Thyme is a natural antiseptic and tonic, and has many medicinal qualities. An herbal tea made from it will help to treat complaints such as a sore throat.

ABOVE *Thyme traditionally symbolizes courage.*

Thyme tea is also good for the treatment of infected gums and mouth ulcers. Further on through the system, thyme helps to relieve indigestion and can improve more severe intestinal symptoms of stomach ulcers. It is also said to be useful for relieving the worst symptoms of hangovers.

Like mint and rosemary, thyme is also a useful treatment for headaches, rheumatism and muscular pain. A few drops of essential oil in a massage oil will help to soothe aching muscles, or you can add a little to the bathwater to ease pain. Thyme is also beneficial as a means of relieving insomnia.

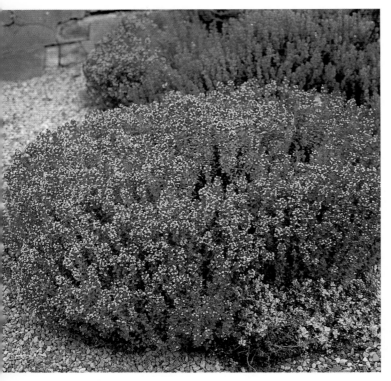

LEFT *Thyme has small, purple flowers and deep green foliage.*

THYME OF DEATH

Thyme has long been associated with death; the sweet-smelling flowers are supposed to harbor the souls of the dead. However, it is often excluded from funeral wreaths on the basis of a tenuous logic that plays on the pun: "death has nothing to do with time," i.e., death is beyond time.

Cooking with Thyme

Thyme is a strong herb that can be added to many winter soups and stews, and helps the body to break down fatty foods during the process of digestion. It is a valuable general flavoring in bouquet garni, which together with parsley and bay leaf is used to flavor soups and stews, and goes very well with game, chicken, fish, and vegetables. It is also a popular ingredient in stuffings and sauces.

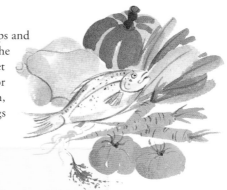

THYME AND PARSLEY STUFFING

This stuffing goes particularly well with lamb.

2 TBL. (30G) BUTTER

½ CUP (50G) FINELY CHOPPED ONIONS

4 TBL. (50G) LARD

½ CUP (100G) WHITE BREAD CRUMBS

1 SMALL EGG, BEATEN

2 TSP. FINELY CHOPPED FRESH THYME

1 TSP. FINELY CHOPPED FRESH PARSLEY

SALT AND BLACK PEPPER

1 Melt the butter in a pan, add the onions and cook until soft but not browned.

2 Add all the remaining ingredients and stir to combine.

3 Use to stuff a leg or shoulder of lamb and bake in the oven for the required time.

ABOVE *Thyme is an extremely versatile herb that can accompany a wide variety of ingredients.*

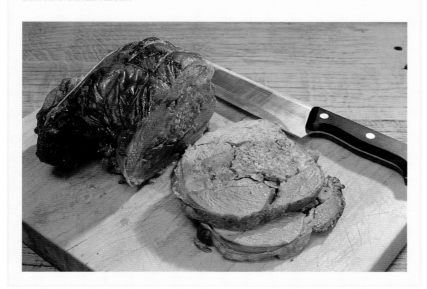

LEFT *Thyme is a perfect ingredient for stuffings to accompany roasts.*

Gemini

MAY 22 – JUNE 21

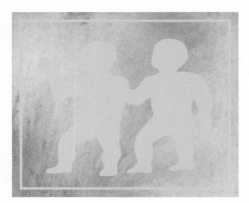

"*MANY GEMINI PERSONS MAY BE SAID TO BE DOUBLE.
ONE TRAIT OF CHARACTER SEEMS TO CONTRADICT
ANOTHER TRAIT.... THEY WANT TO TRAVEL, AND THEY
WANT TO STAY AT HOME. THEY WISH TO STUDY AND THEY
WISH TO PLAY. THEY ARE HAPPY AND UNHAPPY, SATISFIED
AND DISSATISFIED AT THE SAME TIME.*"

ELEANOR KIRK *THE INFLUENCE OF THE
ZODIAC UPON HUMAN LIFE*

The twin stars, Castor and Pollux, were the original heavenly twins recognized as the sign of Gemini. Now associated with the planet Mercury, the most important herbs under Gemini are lavender, vervain, parsley, and caraway. Before finding out about the many qualities of these herbs, it is interesting to look at the way other seasonal herbs play a role in the traditional festivals and rituals that fall under the Gemini dates.

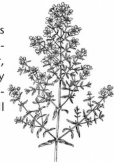

ABOVE *St. John's
wort is the herb
that is most often
associated with the
summer solstice.*

Seasonal Rites

One of the year's most important festivals usually falls on the final day that the sun is in Gemini: the summer solstice on June 21st. This is the longest day of the year and marks the peak of the sun's strength. After the advent of Christianity, many solstice rites were transferred to Midsummer's Day on June 24th, the Christian feast day of St. John the Baptist. The ancient solstice rites were held at dawn on the longest day of the year, to greet the sun, and also at sunset – around the midsummer fire – to wish it well on its receding journey for the rest of the year.

Many herbs are associated with the solstice and should be brought into the house for luck at this time of year. They are incorporated into rituals by using them to decorate the place where the ritual is held. Solstice herbs include yarrow, bird's foot trefoil, larkspur, ragged robin, orpine, lily, wild rose, and wild thyme. But of all the midsummer herbs, the most important by far is St. John's wort.

ABOVE *Wild roses
and ragged robin
are just two among
many solstice herbs.*

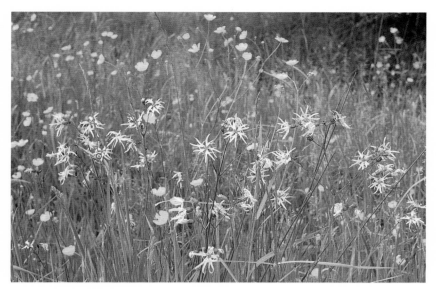

LEFT *A meadow full of mauve- colored ragged robin, in flower during the summer solstice.*

The Solstice Herbs

St. John's wort *(Hypericum perforatum)* flowers at midsummer and has always been used to drive away evil spirits, since nothing can hide from the brightness of the sun. It has bright yellow flowers, with petals that spread out like the rays of the sun. Its leaves, when crushed, emit a smell of incense, and this adds to its ceremonial character. The yellow flowers release a red oil when squeezed, which was thought to be the blood of St. John. A stem of St. John's wort should be hung over the doorway at the solstice to keep evil from the house, and St. John's wort was always burned on solstice bonfires.

Sweet woodruff is another important solstice herb. This flower is scentless until it is dried, when it gains an aroma similar to that of hay. Traditionally, it was used to sweeten the air and encourage good health and luck. Roses and sweet woodruff together used to be made into garlands, which were hung up to attract peace and goodwill. These garlands, which sometimes included ragged robin as well, were called Barnaby garlands because they were hung on St. Barnabas Day. This also falls within the sign of Gemini, on June 11th; before the calendar was changed in 1752, it fell eleven days later, at midsummer.

GEMINI COMPLAINTS

Influenced by Mercury, the Gemini sign rules the lungs, hands, and fingers, and therefore governs complaints such as bronchitis, asthma, the common cold, and even warts and chilblains. It does not necessarily follow that the Gemini herbs are the best remedies for these symptoms – for the most useful herbs to help treat Gemini complaints, *see pages 124–127.*

RIGHT *The Gemini personality is likely to suffer from a lot of colds.*

Lavender

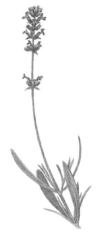

Lavender is first recorded as having been used as a herb by the ancient Greeks and Romans. They added it to their bath water, and its name derives from the Latin *lavare*, meaning to wash. It was the Romans who introduced lavender to Britain in the first century AD. But most people associate lavender with Tudor times, which is when it really started to be used extensively, and began to be grown in domestic gardens.

Healing with Lavender

Lavender is a natural sedative, and its medicinal uses have traditionally been focused on its ability to soothe and calm. Lavender tea (made from an infusion of the flowers) will help to ease many of the symptoms of colds, headaches in particular.

Lavender tea will also help calm nerves, flatulence, dizziness and fainting. Add fresh flowers or essential oil to the bath water to help you to sleep, and use the essential oil in aromatherapy – in a massage oil, or burned on an oil burner – for anxiety and depression. Lavender is also antibacterial in its action, and its oil is a useful remedy for cuts, stings and burns.

BELOW A swathe of lavender brings color as well as scent to this perennial bed.

ABOVE The antibacterial property of lavender makes it ideal for remedying cuts and stings.

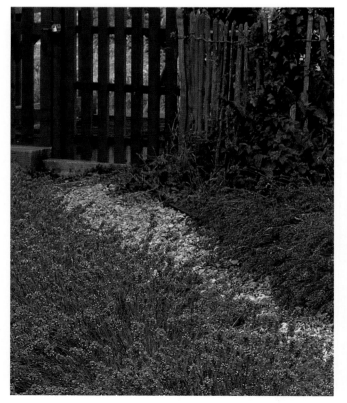

RELAXING POWERS

Lavender was prized for its relaxing properties, and stuffed into cushions it was used to help bring on sleep. People had so much faith in its soporific abilities that it was even believed to make lions and tigers docile.

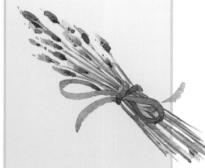

LAVENDER FURNITURE POLISH

Lavender is traditionally used in furniture polish for its cleansing and scented properties.

12 OZ. (350G) BEESWAX

3 PTS. (1.75L) TURPENTINE

2 PTS. (1L) WATER

2 OZ. (50G) SOFT SOAP

FEW DROPS OIL OF LAVENDER

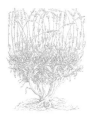

ABOVE *There are many different species of lavender, that generally flower between June and September.*

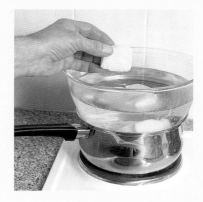

1 Melt the beeswax in the turpentine in a double boiler.

2 In a separate saucepan, boil the water and stir in the soap. Leave both pans to cool.

3 Add the soap and water mixture to the beeswax mixture, stirring slowly and continuously until the combined mixture is the consistency of thick cream.

4 Add lavender oil until the mixture is scented but not pungent.

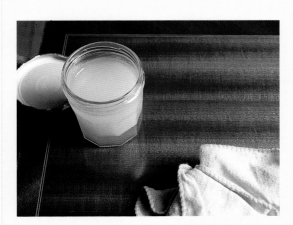

WARNING
Be careful when heating the turpentine as it is highly flammable.

Cooking with Lavender

Lavender is not nearly as popular in cooking as it once was, but the flowers have a delicate flavor that can be used in cookies and in jelly (excellent as an accompaniment to baked meat).

Try mixing lavender flowers with other herbs to use as seasoning for soups and stews; mixed with other chopped fresh herbs, they make an excellent flavoring for types of pork roasts or ham.

Harvesting lavender can be problematic, since lavender plants are a favorite of bees due to their abundant nectar. It is even recommended that lavender is harvested under the cover of darkness.

LEFT *Dried lavender is very decorative and smells sweet.*

HOME-MADE LAVENDER WATER

An old-fashioned preparation, ideal for refreshing the skin, lavender water is easy to make – simply place fresh lavender flowers in a jar with heated spring water, shake to mix well, then leave in a sunny place for a day. Strain into a bottle and store in the refrigerator. Lavender water can be used as a tonic after the skin has been cleansed and before applying moisturizer.

LAVENDER JELLY

you will need:

2 LB. (1KG) GREEN COOKING APPLES

2 PT. (900ML) WATER

2 TBL. WHITE WINE VINEGAR

1 LARGE HANDFUL LAVENDER FLOWERS

1LB. (450G) SUGAR

2 TBL. LEMON JUICE

1 TBL. LAVENDER FLOWERS

1 Chop the apples, including the peel and cores. Put them in a large pan with the water and bring to a boil.

2 Add the vinegar and the handful of lavender flowers and simmer for about 30 minutes, until the mixture is soft and pulpy.

3 Pour the mixture into a jelly bag and let it strain overnight.

4 Next day, measure the juice and allow a pound of sugar per 2½cups

of juice. Add the sugar and bring the mixture to a boil.

5 Continue to boil steadily until the mixture reaches setting point (a teaspoonful put on a cold plate will form a skin quickly).

6 Skim off any scum, then add the lemon juice and 1tbl. of lavender flowers.

7 Let it cool for a few minutes, then pour into jars. Seal the jars when the mixture is cool.

8 Serve with hot or cold meat.

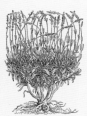

Vervain

This herb was sacred to the ancient Egyptians, Greeks, Romans, and Druids, all of whom used it for ritual purification. Today it is used as a herbal remedy for the treatment of tension, stress, and depression following illness such as the flu or a viral infection. It is a tall plant that reaches 3 feet (1m) high and has delicate pale mauve flowers on spikes. Vervain should be harvested just before the flowers open in July.

RIGHT *Vervain offers a popular herbal treatment for depression and nervous tension.*

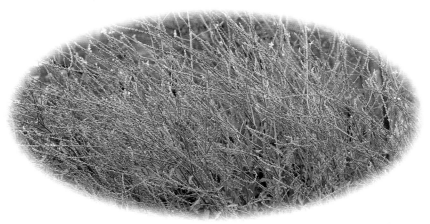

Healing with Vervain

Vervain is used to treat depression, anxiety, and nervous exhaustion, often taken as a tea made from any of the above-ground parts of the plant. The tea is also useful as a general detoxicant to pep up the system. It helps to reduce headaches and migraines, especially those associated with nausea.

Cooking with Vervain

Vervain is not widely used as a culinary plant, since it has to be treated with caution. The chopped leaves have a reputation as an aphrodisiac and can be added to dishes in very small quantities – but take care to use it sparingly.

LEFT *Vervain is spiky in appearance, with small flowers. Only the part of the plant above ground is of use.*

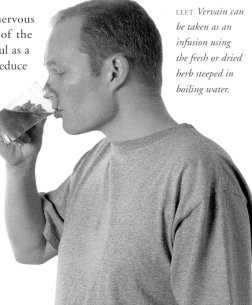

LEFT *Vervain can be taken as an infusion using the fresh or dried herb steeped in boiling water.*

Parsley

$\mathcal{M}$uch loved by cooks for adding flavor and color to dishes, parsley is a welcome sight in kitchen gardens. Easy to grow from seed, it has many useful properties. There are two major types – the familiar curly herb and the flat-leafed variety. Flat-leafed parsley tends to have a stronger flavor than the curly variety.

Healing with Parsley

Parsley is packed with iron, minerals, and vitamins, including Vitamin C. It is excellent for strengthening mother's milk, and for increasing it. It is also a strong diuretic, so it is often used to treat infections of the urinary system. It promotes fresh breath and, since it contains an antiseptic, parsley is also useful as a poultice for applying to stings and cuts.

HERB OF DEATH

Parsley was a herb of death for the Ancient Greeks and was believed to have sprung from the blood of Archemorus, the herald of death. Perhaps for this reason it acquired an association with Satan.

Parsley was, in fact, believed to be the servant of Satan, and one had to go to quite some lengths to grow it safely. First, boiling water had to be poured over the ground as a deterrent to the devil before the seed was sown. Next, you had to be sure to plant it between midday and three o'clock on Good Friday, because the devil is preoccupied at that time. And then, just to be certain it was safe, you had to grow three plants: one for yourself and two for the devil. Moving a parsley plant was even more dangerous, as it heralded a death in the household.

ABOVE *Parsley grows in florets and its bright green color is indicative of its being high in vitamin C.*

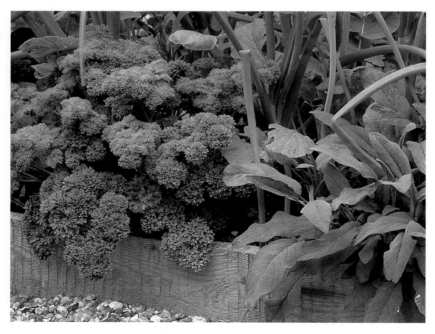

LEFT *Many parts of the parsley plant can be collected and used herbally, from the roots to the flower seeds.*

Cooking with Parsley

Parsley is a staple ingredient in the general flavoring of bouquet garni (which also includes thyme and bay leaf). Its flavor is strong, but can be destroyed by lengthy cooking, so it is always best to add the parsley in the last few minutes. It is also a popular garnish, either finely chopped or in sprigs, where its strong, fresh color adds life and interest to the presentation of food.

Parsley sauce is a popular accompaniment to boiled ham and broiled or fried fish, and parsley is one of the ingredients in *fines herbes*, which is sprinkled on eggs or used in a *fines herbes* omelet. Also included in *fines herbes* are chervil, chives, and tarragon; all should be used in roughly equal quantities and chopped finely.

PARSLEY SAUCE

you will need

2 TBL. (30G) BUTTER

2 TBL. (30G) ALL-PURPOSE FLOUR

2¼ PINT (275ML) MILK

3 15ML TABLESPOONS CHOPPED PARSLEY

SALT AND PEPPER

1 Melt the butter in a saucepan. Add the flour and cook for a minute or two, stirring and taking care not to brown the mixture.

2 Add the milk, a little at a time, stirring thoroughly between each addition.

3 Bring to a boil and add the chopped parsley. Season with salt and pepper to taste, then serve.

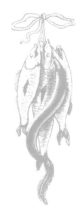

ABOVE *Parsley is often used to bring out the flavor of fish dishes.*

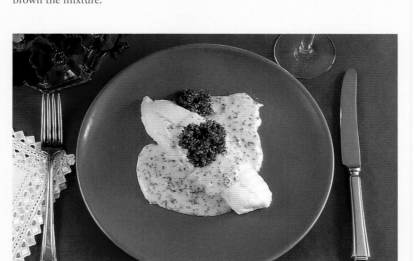

LEFT *Serve broiled or poached cod with parsley sauce as a traditional fish meal.*

Caraway

Caraway is known to have been used in cooking since Stone Age times, and was used as a medicine by the ancient Egyptians to cure colic and other stomach disorders. The plant is related to anise and produces tapered seeds that have a pleasant, slightly pungent aniseed flavor.

Caraway

Caraway combines well with other herbs for the treatment of a variety of problems. Try for example bringing together caraway with the following for effective remedies against diarrhea and bronchitis: agrimony, bayberry, camomile, and white horehound.

Healing with Caraway

Caraway is useful for its digestive properties. You can use the leaves, roots, and seeds, either to eat raw or as an infusion. They will aid digestion, sweeten the breath, and prevent flatulence. Caraway is also useful, if taken just before a meal, for stimulating a poor appetite.

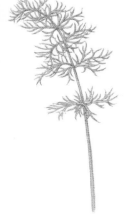

ABOVE *Caraway's medicinal properties are enhanced when combined with other herbs.*

STRAY NOT

In folklore, caraway is believed to prevent things from straying; placed among your possessions it will protect them from thieves, and put into love potions it will prevent a lover from wandering.

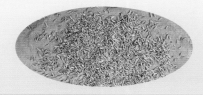

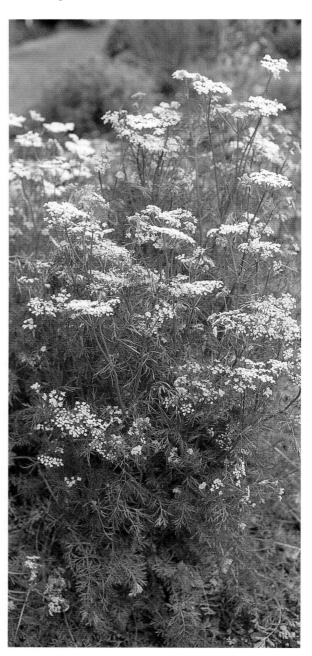

Cooking with Caraway

Caraway has a flavor reminiscent of aniseed. Although you can eat the leaves and the root, it is the seeds that are most commonly used in cooking. They are used in breads, crackers and cakes (caraway seed cake is an obvious example), and the flavor also goes extremely well with cheese. The leaves can be eaten in salads, and the roots boiled or steamed and eaten as a vegetable.

CARAWAY CRACKERS

You will need:

4 TBL. (50G) ALL-PURPOSE FLOUR, SIFTED

2 TBL. (25G) BUTTER

¼ CUP (50G) GRATED CHEDDAR CHEESE

½ TEASPOON CARAWAY SEEDS

½ TEASPOON DIJON MUSTARD

1 EGG YOLK

PINCH OF SALT

1 Put the flour and salt into a bowl and rub in the butter.

2 Add the cheese and caraway seeds and stir in with a knife blade.

3 Lightly beat the egg yolk with the mustard and stir these into the mixture.

4 Add a little cold water if necessary to create a softer dough.

5 Put in a plastic bag and chill for an hour in the refrigerator.

6 Roll the dough out on a floured board until it is about ¼ in. (3mm) thick, and cut out the cookies with a round cutter.

7 Place on a greased cookie sheet and cook in a moderately hot oven (200°C/400°F) for about 7 minutes, until golden brown.

8 Delicious served hot with consommé or cheese.

CARAWAY INFUSION

To make an infusion from the seeds, pour boiling water over three teaspoons of crushed seeds in the bottom of a cup.

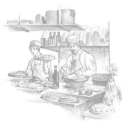

ABOVE *A woodblock print showing busy industry in a baker's kitchen.*

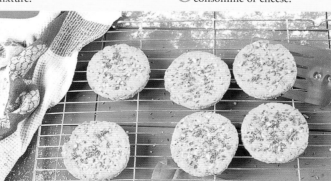

Cancer

JUNE 22 – JULY 22

"THIS SIGN IS CALLED THE PARADOX OF THE TWELVE.... GENERALLY SPEAKING, THE GENIUS OF THE CANCER SIGN IS EXCEEDINGLY DIFFICULT TO EXPLAIN. THOSE BORN UNDER IT HAVE A PERSISTENT WILL, A CLUTCH OF DETERMINATION, INTUITION, AND PURPOSE."

ELEANOR KIRK *THE INFLUENCE OF THE ZODIAC UPON HUMAN LIFE*

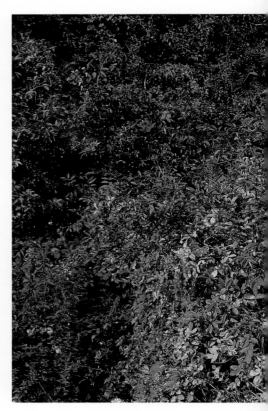

Cancer is ruled by the moon, which represents the feminine principle. The herbs chiefly associated with the sign are agrimony, daisy, and hyssop. These are covered in depth on the following pages, but first it is interesting to look at how seasonal herbs play a role in the traditional festivals and rituals that fall within the Cancer sign.

BELOW *The daisy is one of the herbs associated with the star sign Cancer.*

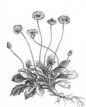

RIGHT *Daisy chains were hung around children's necks to protect them from spirits.*

Seasonal Rites

None of the eight major European festivals fall under the sign of Cancer, but there are also several minor festivals. St. Peter's Day is June 29th, when the rushbearings were traditionally held. This festival involved loading carts with rushes and taking them in procession to churches where the rushes would be used as a floor covering.

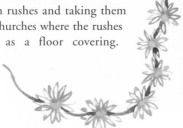

Although rushes were a traditional floor covering, this festival raised the practice to a ceremonial level.

The rushcarts were transported and unloaded ceremonially, and were decorated with herb garlands containing roses, St. John's wort, and vervain. Roses are sacred to the Virgin Mary, St. John's wort is the ancient herb of the sun, and vervain is a ritual cleansing herb whose use dates back to the Celts, although the Celts would never have picked it before the "dog days" of early July, after the dog star first rises.

July 5th is the old Midsummer's Day (before the calendar change of 1752), and is a time when Robin Goodfellow, or Puck, is likely to lead people astray. To guard against this, people traditionally carried a protective herb such as St. John's wort, or a stick of rowan. Children were protected by daisy chains around their necks; the daisy is another flower of the sun, since it only opens during the day.

BELOW *Rosehips bring a dash of bright red to this hedge during fall.*

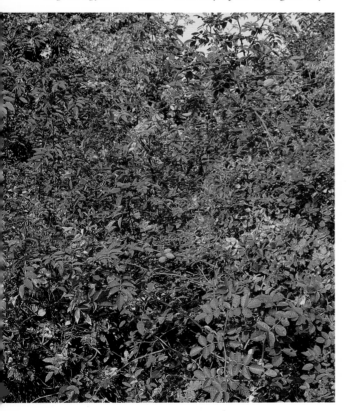

CANCER COMPLAINTS

Through the ruling influence of the moon, Cancer governs the feminine parts of the body most associated with motherhood: the womb and the breast. The illnesses and complaints Cancer governs include menstrual problems, breastfeeding problems, childbirth, and menopause. Popular herbs for treating these complaints are motherwort, raspberry leaf, and evening primrose. It does not necessarily follow that the Cancer herbs are the right choice for treating these problems – for the best herbs to help relieve these symptoms, see pages 124-127.

LEFT *Cancerians are governed by the moon and are affected by problems associated with motherhood.*

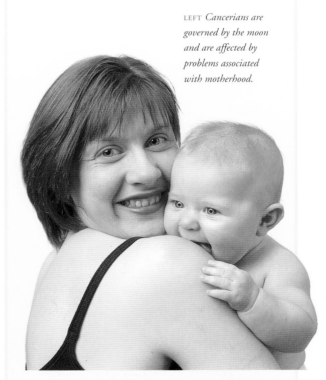

Agrimony

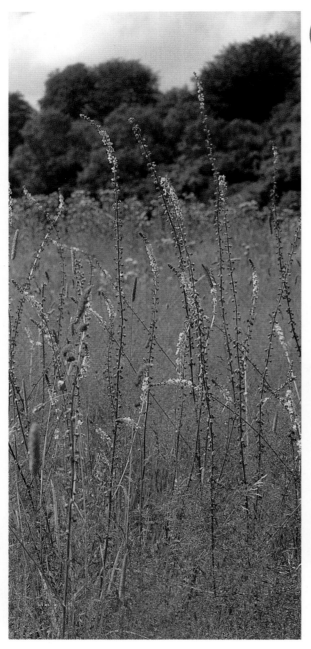

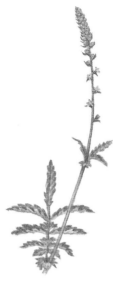

grimony commonly grows by the roadside in European countries and was introduced to the U.S. by the early settlers. It carries many five-pointed yellow flowers up the stem in summer, followed by little burrs in the fall. Agrimony used to be popular for dyeing wool. This plant was widely used as a medicinal herb in ancient Persia, Greece, and Rome. The word agrimony comes from the Greek *argemon*, meaning a disorder of the eye. Originally, agrimony was famous for its ability to heal wounds and was used especially for eye injuries and complaints.

ABOVE *Agrimony is a multipurpose herb that can be used to treat a whole host of ailments.*

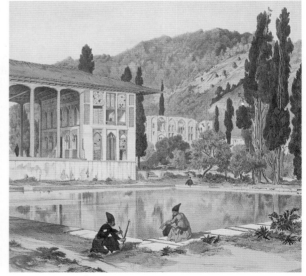

LEFT *Agrimony grows in abundance in the wild and has many practical as well as herbal uses, from dyeing wool to healing wounds.*

ABOVE *Ancient Persia, shown here in a painting by Jules Laurens, was one of the first nations to use agrimony for medicinal purposes.*

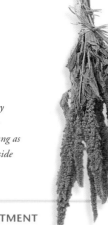

RIGHT *To dry agrimony, it should be hung as a bunch, upside down.*

Healing with Agrimony

Agrimony has antibiotic, astringent, and anti-inflammatory qualities; it contains tannin among other things. It is particularly good for treating the problem of excessive bleeding during menstruation.

The dried plant is infused to make a tea that is helpful in treating sore throats and coughs, diarrhea (especially in children), peptic ulcers, and cystitis. It is a diuretic as well as an astringent, which is why it is so effective in treating any complaints that include bleeding from the urinary tract – although you should always see a doctor for any such complaint before applying self-diagnosed herbal remedies.

True to its original use in ancient Persia, agrimony is also excellent as an eyewash for treating conjunctivitis. Use a cooled infusion in an eyecup, or hold a cold compress against the eye.

A TREATMENT FOR EARACHE

Agrimony leaves can be used to treat the type of earache caused by a build-up of wax.

Make a weak infusion of the leaves (see page 17) and use a dropper to apply it to the ears several times a day. The infusion should be warmed for effective treatment. Continue applying the infusion until the pain and discomfort eases.

Cooking with Agrimony

Agrimony has never been used as a culinary herb, although the infused tea, which is generally taken for medicinal purposes, has a pleasant apricot scent.

DEATHLY SLEEP

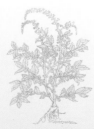

Agrimony was also believed to have strange powers that affected sleeping patterns. Folklore has it that if a sprig of agrimony was placed under the pillow of a person about to lay down their head, they would fall into such a deep sleep that they would appear dead. Absolutely nothing would wake them unless the agrimony was removed from under the pillow.

WOOL DYEING

Depending on the mordant (fixative) used, the color it produces will vary.

For every 4 oz. (100g) of mordanted wool you will need 7oz. (200g) of agrimony, using any above-ground parts of the plant.

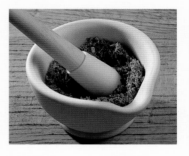

1 Crush the plant.

2 Simmer in just enough water to cover for 3 hours.

3 Strain and cool the liquid.

4 Add the wetted wool to this liquid and bring to a boil over an hour, then simmer for another hour.

5 Rinse the wool in hot, then warm, and then cold water, and dry. A chrome mordant gives a fawn color; iron will give brownish gray.

Daisy

Small daisies, with their delicate white petals and sunny faces, are a familiar sight during the summer months, when they grow in abundance over grassy areas. The word "daisy," means "day's eye," a name given to this flower because it opens its petals in the sun and closes them up at night. It is sometimes said that daisies are the true harbingers of spring, and it isn't spring until you can "plant your foot on a dozen daisies."

FLOWER OF LOVE

Daisies were often associated with love, and it is still a custom for girls to pull off the petals one at a time reciting "he loves me, he loves me not" or "tinker, tailor, soldier, sailor, rich man, poor man, beggar man, thief."

Healing with Daisy

One of our most common plants, daisy is a traditional cure for wounds and bruises; one of its common names is "bruise-wort." If you crush the leaves and hold them against a bruise they will help to reduce the swelling. The leaves can be eaten fresh or infused into a tea; the flowers are also edible.

The flowers are more commonly used in tea, which makes a good treatment for diarrhea or for coughs and colds, and it helps to relieve aches such as arthritis, rheumatism, liver and kidney problems, and backache. You can add an infusion to the bathwater as a direct tonic for the skin and to help ease persistent backache.

ABOVE *The daisy is valued by herbalists who use its flowers in infusions to treat coughs and catarrh.*

RIGHT *The daisy is often dotted across lawns and meadows, and although some gardeners consider the plant to be a weed, it has several herbal uses.*

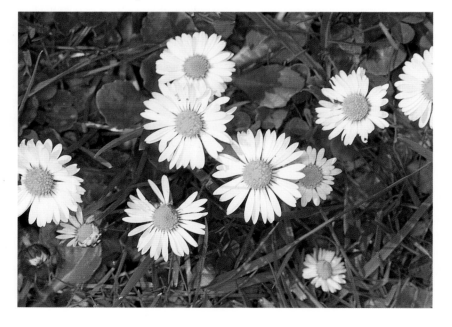

Cooking with Daisy

Daisy is not used widely in cooking, but the young leaves and flowers can be eaten in salads, and because they are so decorative you can use them as an attractive garnish for all sorts of dishes, especially cakes and cold desserts.

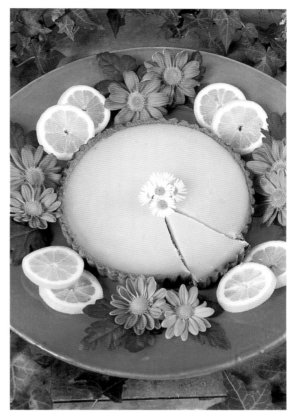

DAISY INFUSION

To make an infusion of daisy leaves, follow the directions on page 16. Add this to a warm bath as a skin tonic or to relieve aching joints.

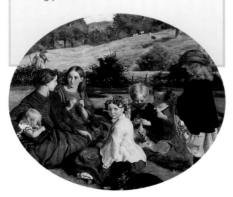

RIGHT This country scene depicts children at play making daisy chains.

ABOVE Daisies can add a final touch as a garnish on desserts.

DAISY CHAINS

The daisy has always symbolized innocence and is associated with children. The tradition of making daisy chains used to be more than just a game; a daisy chain worn around a child's neck protected it from being carried away by the fairies – the influence of the sun would ward off the darker forces. It was important that the chain was joined at both ends – to create an unbroken circle with no gap for evil spirits to enter through.

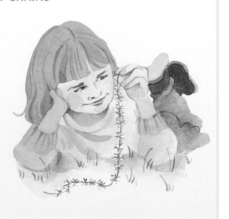

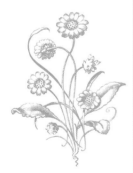

ABOVE The daisy is abundant, growing on lawns and in meadows everywhere.

Hyssop

yssop originates from central and southern Europe and western Asia, and was used by the ancient civilizations of the Middle East and the Mediterranean. The word has remained almost unchanged from the Hebrew name for the plant, *esob*, which is referred to several times in the Old Testament. Psalm 51, verse 7, says "Purge me with hyssop and I shall be clean."

ANTIBIOTIC EFFECT

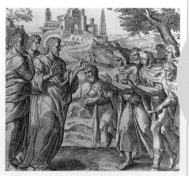

ABOVE *This painting depicts Jesus healing lepers.*

There is some dispute as to whether the plant manifested in the Old Testament was the same plant we now call hyssop, but current thinking is that it most probably was. Apart from anything else, the mold that produces penicillin grows on hyssop leaves, and using this to bathe people would have an antibiotic effect; lepers were bathed in an infusion of hyssop.

WARNING
Hyssop should not be taken during pregnancy, or by anyone who is highly strung.

Healing with Hyssop

Hyssop is infused and drunk as a remedy for respiratory complaints such as coughs, asthma, bronchitis, and rhinitis. Applied as a compress or an essential oil it helps to heal burns, wounds, and bruises.

ABOVE *The delicate hyssop is used to remedy a wide range of complaints.*

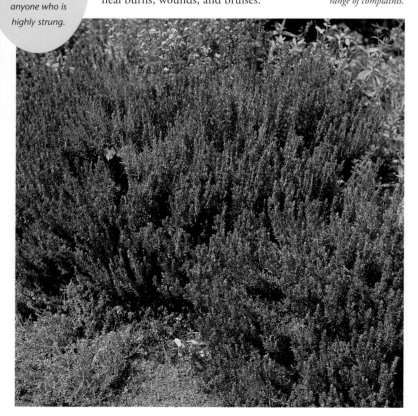

RIGHT *Hyssop has long been used as an herb in Europe, especially in Mediterranean countries, and in the Middle East.*

Cooking with Hyssop

Hyssop has a strong flavor, reminiscent of mint, and is delicious in cooking, but should be used carefully as the taste is very strong. The leaves help the system to digest fatty foods. Hyssop flowers are edible, and are most useful tossed in salads to add visual interest; the flowers come in shades of blue, pink, or white.

Hyssop goes particularly well with game, lamb, sausages, and variety meat, and is good in rich terrines and patès, and stuffings; the chopped leaves are wonderful in a steak and kidney pie. With roast beef, you can add hyssop to Yorkshire pudding batter. In parts of France it is used as a standard ingredient in bouquet garni, and the flavor also marries well with tomatoes in soups and stews.

A few finely chopped hyssop leaves in a fruit pie help to bring out the flavor of orchard fruits, and you can add a couple of sprigs of hyssop to a sugar syrup for a fruit salad. Add the hyssop to the sugar and water mix during the boiling stage, and remove it before pouring the syrup over the fruit.

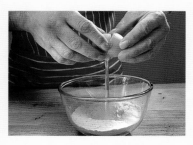

HYSSOP YORKSHIRE PUDDING

1 CUP (100G) ALL-PURPOSE FLOUR

PINCH OF SALT

1 EGG

1¼ CUPS (275ML) MILK

1 TSP. FINELY CHOPPED HYSSOP

2 TBL. (30G) SHORTENING

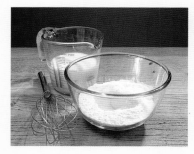

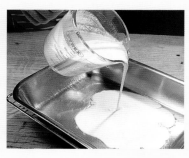

1 Preheat the oven to 220C/425F.

2 Sift the flour and salt into a bowl and make a well in the center. Break the egg into the well and add half the milk.

3 Whisk the egg and milk together, gradually incorporating the flour from around the edge. Whisk in the remaining milk, a little at a time.

4 Add the chopped hyssop to the batter and leave the mixture to rest for a few minutes.

5 Put the fat (preferably dripping from around the meat) in the bottom of a shallow, 6-in. (17cm) pan and heat in the oven for 3–4 minutes.

6 Remove the pan from the oven and pour the batter mixture into it. Return to the oven for 15 minutes. Serve.

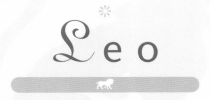

Leo

JULY 23 – AUGUST 23

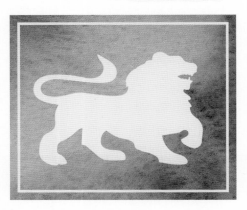

"KIND HEARTED, GENEROUS, SYMPATHETIC, AND MAGNETIC.... THEY ARE EMOTIONAL, VERY INTUITIVE, AND ARE GENERALLY ABLE BY MEANS OF THIS POWER TO ESCAPE THE CONSEQUENCES OF THEIR ACTIONS."

ELEANOR KIRK *THE INFLUENCE OF THE ZODIAC UPON HUMAN LIFE*

Leo, which comes from the Latin word meaning lion, is ruled by the sun. The key herbs of Leo are bay, camomile, poppy, and rue. Before discovering more about the qualities of these herbs, it is interesting to look at the festivals and rituals traditionally held at this time of the year.

Seasonal Rites

August 1st is the ancient Celtic feast of Lughnasadh, held in honor of the great god Lug. This celebration has been Christianized as Lammas – or loaf-mass – to mark the beginning of the harvest period. The earliest recorded version of the festival took the form of a frenzied circle dance and the miming of plowing, cobbling, tanning, spinning, and weaving – all performed in the hope of guaranteeing a good harvest. Of all the herbs that grow at this time of year, the poppy is the one most strongly associated with the harvest. The poppy is often seen growing in and around fields of grain, bringing a little color to the landscape.

Corn Dolly

Traditionally, the spirit of the grain resided in the fields. It was believed that when the grain came to be reaped at harvest time, the spirit was driven back until eventually it was forced to hide in the last remaining section of wheat. Since no one wanted to be the one to destroy the grain spirit's last refuge, the reapers used to take turns to throw their sickles at it until the last of the grain was cut. These stalks were then gathered

LEFT *The bright red color of the poppy decorates meadows and fields in August.*

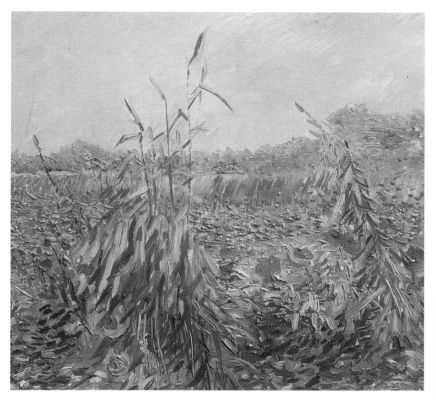

LEFT *In this oil painting by Vincent Van Gogh, the bright flowers of poppies are scattered among green stalks of wheat after the harvest has been reaped.*

BELOW *A corn dolly was made by rural communities each harvest time to represent the spirit of the grain.*

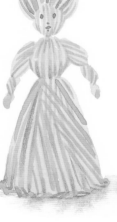

LEO COMPLAINTS

Ruled by the sun, the sign of Leo governs the heart. It is appropriate that the heart of the solar system – the sun – should rule the literal heart of our own bodies. So Leo influences illnesses and diseases of the blood and the circulation. These include varicose veins, hemorrhoids, high blood pressure, low blood pressure, anemia, and poor circulation. It does not necessarily follow that the Leo herbs are the most appropriate for treating the complaints coming under this sign – for the best herbs to treat Leo symptoms, *see pages 124–127.*

and made into a corn dolly, which would be seated in the place of honor at the Lughnasadh feast.

The corn dolly, which represented the spirit of the grain, would be preserved over the winter and then plowed back into the fields the following spring. The corn spirit was sometimes said to take the form of a great cat, known as the corn cat. Instead of making a corn dolly, the Celts would often sacrifice a cat. This ritual became tamer eventually, and in many places today a cat is chosen to be decorated with ribbons for the day.

LEFT *Those born under the sign of Leo are prone to suffer from illnesses or diseases that are linked to blood and circulation.*

Bay

Bay originated in southern Europe, although it is now grown the world over. It was sacred to the Greek god Apollo, whose priestesses consumed large quantities of it before declaring the pronouncements of his oracle at Delphi. They may have been helped along by the narcotic effect that bay has in high doses. Bay is best known, however, for its association with the Romans, who made wreaths of it – laurel wreaths – to crown their great poets and victorious athletes. The Latin name, *Laurus nobilis*, comes from the words *laurus* meaning "praise" and *nobilis* meaning "renowned."

BELOW *Bay trees in containers are popular in terrace and balcony gardens.*

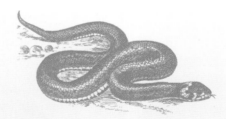

ABOVE *The leaves of the bay shrub, popular for flavoring food, are harvested in late summer.*

Healing with Bay

Bay is known to stimulate the appetite and helps to ease the digestion; it is generally taken as an infusion. A few drops of the essential oil in a carrier massage oil – such as almond, grapeseed, or apricot kernel oil – can be rubbed onto problematic joints to reduce rheumatic pain.

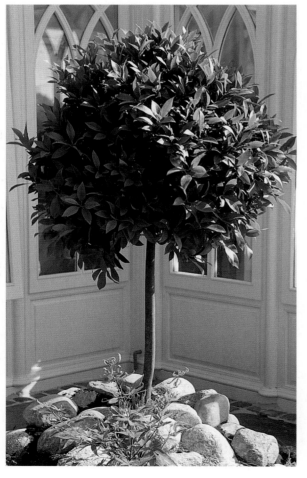

BAY THE GUARDIAN

ABOVE *Bay is believed to protect against snakebite.*

In more recent folklore, bay became so associated with the good and the honorable that it was credited with protecting against disease, snakebite, witchcraft, and most other evils. Shepherds would wear a sprig of bay under their caps to guard them against lightning.

Cooking with Bay

Bay is one of the standard ingredients of bouquet garni, along with parsley and thyme, which forms a general flavoring for all manner of soups and stews. Fresh bay leaves taste stronger than dried ones, although dried bay is still worth using since it holds its flavor well. Use it in stocks, soups, stews, and marinades, and add it to the liquid in which you poach fish. You can remove the leaf before serving.

You can also keep a bay leaf in your rice canister to flavor the rice, especially if you use it in Mediterranean or oriental dishes.

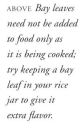

ABOVE *Bay leaves need not be added to food only as it is being cooked; try keeping a bay leaf in your rice jar to give it extra flavor.*

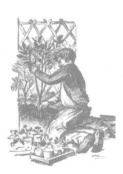

ABOVE *Bay Laurel thrives in coastal gardens and can grow to a height of 18 ft. (5.5 m).*

BOUQUET GARNI

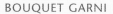

2 SPRIGS OF THYME

3 SPRIGS OF PARSLEY

1 BAY LEAF

6 PEPPERCORNS

1 GREEN LEAF OF A LEEK

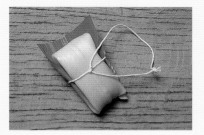

2 Take a piece of string about 10–12 in. (25–30 cm) in length and tie one end around the package so the contents are secure.

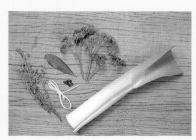

1 Place the herbs and peppercorns on the leek leaf, then fold the leaf around them to make a package.

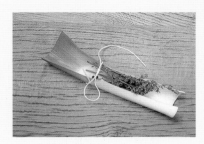

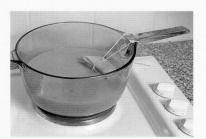

3 Place the bouquet garni in the stock, soup, or stew, and tie the end of the string to the handle of the pan, so you can retrieve it easily.

4 Remove and discard the bouquet garni from the cooked food.

Camomile

This herb has been widely used since the time of the ancient Egyptians, and it is still used to make one of the most popular of all herbal teas. Its name is a reference to its scent, since it comes from the Greek and means "apple on the ground"; all parts of the plant smell strongly of apple.

ABOVE *The list of uses for camomile is lengthy, but it is particularly well known for its sedative properties.*

Healing with Camomile

Camomile has strong antiseptic and anti-inflammatory properties. It is generally taken as an infusion to treat mouth ulcers, sore gums, and peptic ulcers.

Camomile is also known to improve the appetite and aid the digestive system. For external treatment, a cold compress is useful in treating wounds, burns, and eczema. Camomile can also be used in an eye wash for eye infections.

WARNING

High doses of camomile can cause both vomiting and vertigo.

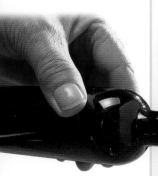

ABOVE *Camomile can also be used in oil and added to baths or used during massage treatments.*

RELAXING OIL

Aromatic oils have been in use for thousands of years, especially in the Middle and Far East. They are commonly used in ayurvedic medicine, a traditional Indian system dating back to 1000 B.C. To make camomile oil, tightly pack a jar with flower heads and cover them with a pure oil such as olive oil. Leave the jar in the sun for 2–3 weeks, then strain the oil. Add a few drops to the bathwater at night to help you relax.

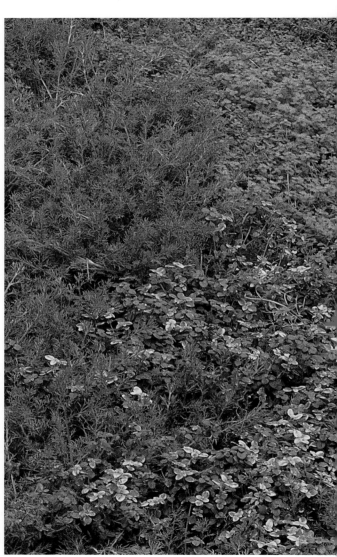

Camomile has long been used as a sedative to calm the nerves and promote healthy sleep; it is often given at bedtime to children who are prone to nightmares. Peter Rabbit, created by writer and artist Beatrix Potter, famously drank camomile tea after having rather too many adventures in Mr. MacGregor's garden.

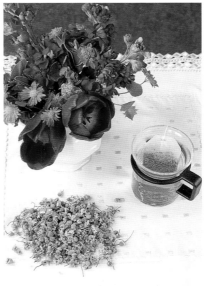

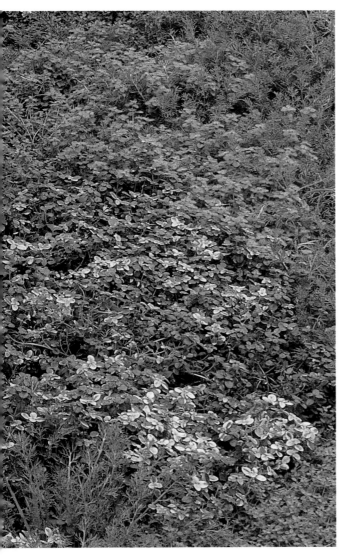

LEFT *Camomile flower heads should be gathered between May and August when they are not wet with dew or rain. They should be dried, but not at a high temperature.*

Cooking with Camomile

Camomile is not used as a culinary herb, although many people drink camomile tea for pleasure as much as for medicinal purposes, often with a little honey added to sweeten it.

Camomile teabags can be bought at supermarkets and grocery stores and the tea drunk in the same way as if you made it with fresh camomile. You can also add camomile teabags to your bath to relax you and to ease any sore or dry skin conditions.

CAMOMILE COMPANION

Camomile has long been used as a companion plant; it has the ability to revive other ailing plants when it is planted near them. It also helps to repel flying insects and, if planted near onions, it is said to improve the crop yield.

Poppy

ield poppies have always been associated with wheatfields, since the seeds need light to germinate, and therefore grow abundantly on land which is plowed – as the soil is turned, so the seeds are exposed to the light. This is why the fields of Flanders, which were churned up in the fighting during World War I, were covered with poppies after the fighting ceased. The poppy became a symbol of remembrance of those killed in battle, and poppies have been worn on Remembrance, or Armistice, Day ever since.

Healing with Poppy

Poppy seedheads are the source of opium – specifically derived from opium poppies (*Papaver somniferum*). A tincture of opium, known as laudanum, was very popular in the 18th and 19th centuries as a painkiller and sedative. Although it was sold widely and taken by men, women, and children alike, it was highly addictive. Opium derivatives, including morphine, are still widely used as a highly effective painkiller, but they are potentially lethal and should only be administered by trained medical staff.

Poppy leaves are said to make a good poultice to hold next to the ear to relieve earache.

ABOVE *The poppy is infamous as the source of opium.*

ABOVE *Earache can be eased with the help of a poultice made of poppy leaves.*

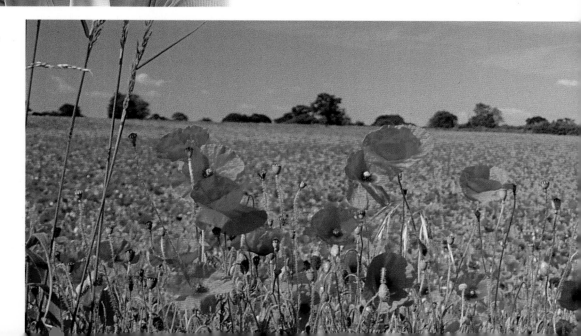

Cooking with Poppy

Poppy seeds can be used in cooking; the ripe seeds of opium poppies are the only nontoxic part of the plant, and both these and the seeds of field poppies can be used. If you collect your own seeds, it is important to make sure they are fully ripe or they will develop mold in storage.

Poppy seeds have a slightly nutty flavor and are delicious sprinkled on crackers, cakes and bread. An oil can be extracted from poppy seeds, which adds a pleasant nutty flavor to cooking.

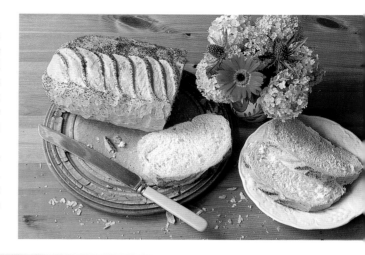

ABOVE *Poppy seeds make a delicious addition to freshly baked bread – simply scatter them over the unbaked dough before it goes in the oven.*

SOPORIFIC POPPY

Poppies are associated with sleep, and legend tells how the Roman god of sleep, Somnus, created the poppy to send Ceres to sleep. Ceres was the goddess of the harvest, but she was so exhausted that the crops were failing without her strength. The poppies, intermingled with the grain, sent Ceres to sleep for the winter, and she awoke refreshed in the spring to bless the following year's crop.

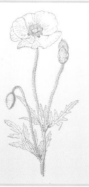

RIGHT *The Greek myth about the poppy links it with sleep and the seasons.*

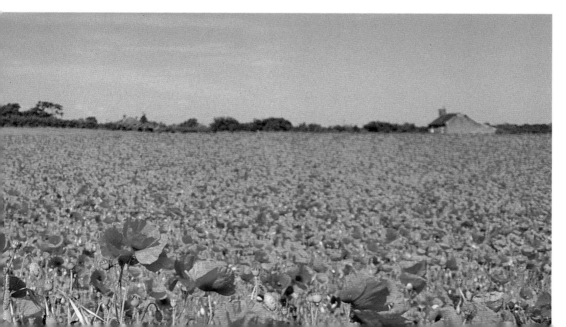

LEFT *Poppies grow in abundance on land that has been plowed and often find their way onto cultivated land.*

69 ☽

Rue

Rue has been incorporated into the medical traditions of numerous cultures, from Europe to China and North America. It has been used as a cure for all kinds of illnesses and diseases, including being used by the ancients as a poison antidote.

Rue has deep spiritual properties, and it is claimed to improve both the eyesight and the inner creative visionary powers. It was one of the most important herbs used against the plague, and because of its strong, incenselike smell, branches of rue were used to sprinkle holy water before the altar. It was used for strewing to help keep away both the plague and other evil influences.

It is also claimed that chewing rue stops you from talking in your sleep, and that ammunition that has been boiled in an infusion of rue always hits its target.

ABOVE *The herb Rue is the subject of many stories and legends concerning its mythical qualities.*

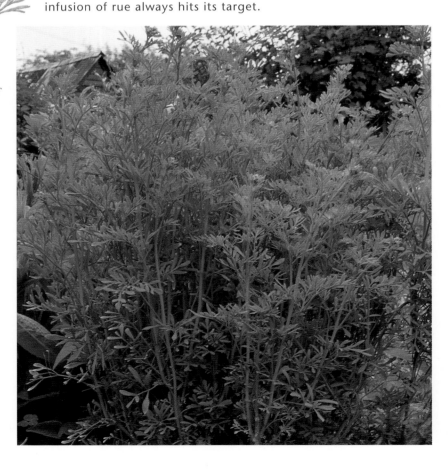

LEFT *Rue has been a popular herb in the long tradition of Chinese herbal medicine.*

Healing with Rue

Rue leaves are infused as a tea, which tastes extremely bitter and usually needs to be sweetened with honey or sugar to be palatable. It is, however, highly valuable as a medicine for the treatment of nervous headaches, high blood pressure, and palpitations.

Rue is useful as a source of iron and helps to harden bones and teeth. Apart from stimulating the appetite, it eases colic and expels worms. It also helps to bring on menstruation. You can use the leaves in a compress to treat wounds, burns, and skin ulcers.

WARNING

Some people suffer serious burns as a reaction to contact with rue, so be careful when you handle the plant. Children in particular can be susceptible. Rue should not be taken during pregnancy.

RUE THE DAY

Rue, as its name indicates, is associated with regret for the past. Also known as "herb of grace," it is a symbol of repentance and regret. It was often used to curse people, by throwing it at their feet to make sure they would "rue the day." However, its strong smell also wards off evil spirits, and a sprig of rue in the pocket, or a plant of it outside the door, provides protection from harm.

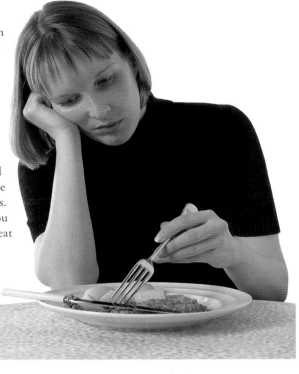

Cooking with Rue

Rue is not often used in cooking, as its taste is very bitter. However, its pungent, incense-like quality can add an unusual twist to fish, egg or cheese recipes if you use the leaf sparingly, in very small quantities.

A strained infusion of the seed harvested from flower heads can also be added to sauces that usually accompany strongly flavored meat and game.

ABOVE *Rue can be used to stimulate a poor appetite, despite its bitter taste.*

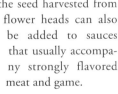

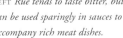

LEFT *Rue tends to taste bitter, but can be used sparingly in sauces to accompany rich meat dishes.*

Virgo

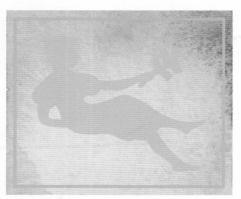

AUGUST 24 – SEPTEMBER 23

"It may be said they maintain their cool and dignified attitude and often impressive presence at the expense of an ill-deserved reputation for coldness of feeling; and thus their nature is rarely, if ever, seen."

HERBERT T. WAITE *COMPENDIUM OF NATAL ASTROLOGY*

The planet Mercury rules Virgo, and the herbs associated with the sign are fennel, southernwood, and valerian. Before looking at these herbs in detail, it is interesting to know a little about the seasonal festivals and rituals that traditionally fall under Virgo.

ABOVE *The herb Valerian is chiefly associated with the star sign of Virgo.*

RIGHT *Virgo is the first astrological sign of the fall.*

Seasonal Rites

The annual autumnal equinox falls on September 22nd or 23rd, just before the sun leaves Virgo. This is the opposite festival to the spring equinox; once again, day and night are equal in length, but this time the days are about to start growing shorter and the nights are becoming longer. The autumn equinox heralds the last few days of the harvest, and looks back at the summer and ahead to the coming winter.

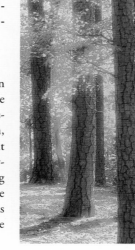

The autumn equinox is therefore all about balance and harmony, and is a time of thought rather than action. Traditional autumn equinox rituals involved giving thanks for the fruits of the summer and meditating on what had been gathered, spiritually as well as literally, to sustain people through the following winter. The sense of balance was accentuated in autumn equinox rituals in which men and women who celebrated the festival faced each other, or moved in circles around each other. The fruits of the harvest gathered at this time of year were celebrated in balance by drinking both white and red wine.

Fruits, nuts, and berries were traditionally gathered in ritual fashion and blessed at the autumn equinox. Late August and September are the months of the year for blackberries, rose hips, elderberries, crab apples, sloes, various kinds of nuts, and rowan berries from the countryside, as well as for cultivated fruit from the garden.

Southernwood, the Virgo herb, is an important cleansing herb for rituals enacted during this time of year. Bundles of dried sticks of Southernwood can be gathered and tied together and burned on a fire. When smoldering, they release a strong, apple-scented smoke that will perfume a building and cleanse it in preparation for the coming of the new season.

ABOVE *The last fruits of summer, such as plums, blackberries, and apples, can still be gathered during the Virgo sign.*

LEFT *Although Virgo's ruling planet Mercury encourages intellectualism, it can result in neuroses.*

VIRGO COMPLAINTS

Mercury, Virgo's ruling planet, has a stimulating, intellectual influence. However, it does have a tendency to be argumentative and even neurotic, and these are traits which often show up in Virgoans. Virgo traditionally rules the digestive system, which is often subject to conditions caused by stress and worry. It is not surprising, therefore, that Virgo governs all stomach complaints, from indigestion and nausea to ulcers, colitis, constipation, diarrhea, and diverticulosis.

It does not necessarily follow, however, that the Virgoan herbs are the most suitable remedies for these conditions – for the best herbs to treat Virgo complaints, see pages 124–127.

RIGHT
Southernwood gives off a pleasant aroma when it is burned.

73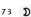

Fennel

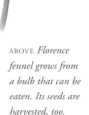

ennel was named from the Latin for "little hay," because of the appearance of the dried leaves. It has been used in cooking for over two thousand years. Although the stems used to be the most popular part of the plant to eat, nowadays it is the seeds that are most used in cooking for their strong flavor.

ABOVE Florence fennel grows from a bulb that can be eaten. Its seeds are harvested, too.

Healing with Fennel

BELOW Fennel, with its fernlike leaves, is a popular culinary herb. Romans used fennel to suppress their appetites.

Fennel has a taste similar to aniseed and is excellent for treating the digestion, and helps to ease constipation, indigestion, and heartburn. The best way to take it is as a tea made from about a teaspoonful of seeds in a cup, infused and then strained. You can also use this tea to ease colic in babies; about a teaspoon is the right dose. Fennel tea is also a traditional treatment for stimulating the flow of breast milk. The eyes, too, are supposed to benefit from fennel; a warm compress will soothe any inflammation of the eye, or a cooled infusion can be used to wash the infected eye.

Recent research has suggested that fennel may also help reduce the toxic effects of alcohol – try drinking a cup before retiring to bed if you think you may have overindulged.

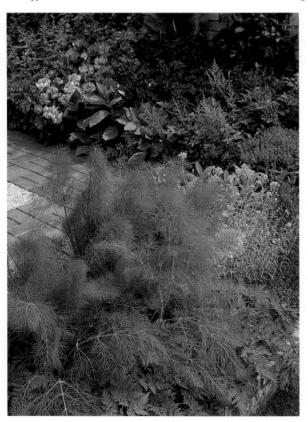

QUELLING HUNGER

One quality of fennel is that it stops you from feeling hungry. It was taken by Roman women as an appetite suppressant to prevent them from becoming overweight, and in puritan communities in North America fennel seeds were known as "meeting seeds" because they were eaten during long church services to quell hunger pangs.

Another (dubious) claim for fennel was that snakes ate it before they shed their skins, to restore their youth.

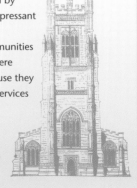

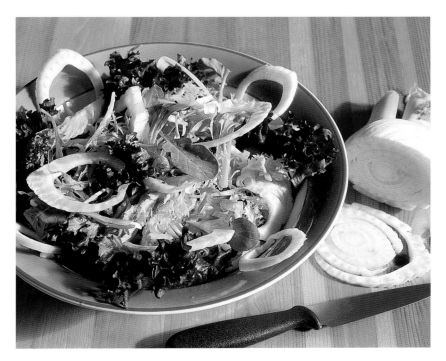

LEFT *Chopped fennel – from either the bulb or the stalk – is a wonderful addition to salad.*

Cooking with Fennel

Fennel is an excellent culinary herb, with a wide range of uses. The seeds and leaves are used chiefly for flavoring, while the stems and bulb can be used as a vegetable either raw or cooked. There are two main varieties of fennel: garden fennel (which also comes in a bronze variety); and Florence fennel, which is grown as an annual and harvested for its delicious bulbous stalk base.

Fennel has a mildly aniseed flavor that goes particularly well with fish. You can use the seeds in sauces, with fish, and sprinkled on bread. Since they are the only part of the plant that keeps well through the winter, they are also very good in winter stews – or let them sprout and use the sprouts in winter salads.

Fennel leaves are fine and feathery, and can be used finely chopped (the easiest way to do this is to shred them with a pair of scissors) to flavor salads, soups, or even cooked vegetables such as carrots. The whole leaves also make a very attractive garnish, and are a little more original and interesting than the ubiquitous parsley sprig. The stems of fennel are most often eaten raw in salads, but you can also cook them with other vegetables such as leeks or celery.

Florence fennel bulbs are considered a great delicacy, with a particularly crunchy texture and a mild aniseed flavor. You can slice them or grate them into salads, often using them as the main ingredient. You can also cook fennel bulbs whole, much as you would cook onions – either boiled, sautéed as a base for stews, or baked. Fennel can be use to flavor jellies made for the purpose of accompanying meat; see the recipe for lavender jelly on page 48.

FENNEL WITH CHEESE SAUCE

4 BULBS OF FLORENCE FENNEL

2 TBL. (30G) BUTTER

2 TBL. (30G) ALL-PURPOSE FLOUR

1¼ CUPS (275ML) MILK

1CUP (100G) MATURE CHEDDAR
CHEESE, GRATED

1 TSP. DIJON MUSTARD

PINCH OF NUTMEG

SALT AND BLACK PEPPER TO SEASON

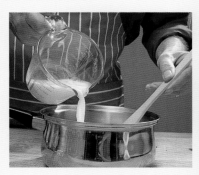

4 Gradually add the milk, stirring well after each addition, to prevent the sauce from becoming lumpy.

5 Add the grated cheese and Dijon mustard and stir until the cheese is thoroughly melted and combined. Season with the nutmeg and salt and pepper to taste.

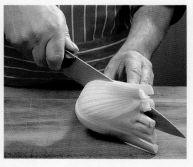

1 Trim and halve the four Florence fennel bulbs.

2 Steam for 20–30 minutes until the vegetable is tender.

3 Meanwhile, melt the butter in a pan. Add the flour and cook for a minute or two, stirring.

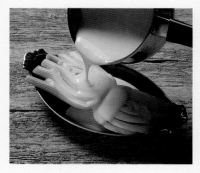

6 Arrange the fennel in a serving dish and pour the cheese sauce over it. Serve hot.

Valerian

Valerian is such an important medicinal herb that its name means "to be healthy." The root is the part chiefly used, and was employed by the Persians, the Chinese, and the Scandinavians centuries ago. Its common names include "all heal," "set all," "cut finger," and "cat's valerian." This last name derives from the fact that both cats and rats are strongly attracted to the scent of valerian root. It is not used for culinary purposes.

PIED PIPER

An explanation of the folk story of the Pied Piper of Hamelin suggests that the piper carried valerian root in his pocket, and it was this, more than the music that he played, which attracted the rats to follow him away from the town.

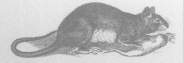

ABOVE *Valerian is said to attract rats, although it is more commonly used as a "cure-all" medicinal herb.*

Healing with Valerian

Valerian is a calmative, and almost all its medicinal uses are associated with its ability to calm the nervous system. A decoction of valerian root – or dried valerian root – can be drunk as a sedative to treat nervous exhaustion and emotional upsets. Although valerian is traditionally used as a sedative, there is some evidence that it acts as a stimulant to people suffering from fatigue.

Another function of Valerian affects the heart: Valerian is thought to strengthen the heart, and can reduce blood pressure. It is a healing herb of many uses; a tincture is even reported to cure dandruff. A decoction is also helpful in treating headaches, insomnia, and intestinal cramps. A poultice of valerian root is a traditional treatment for wounds and cuts, which explains its common name, "cut finger."

Valerian (*Valeriana officinalis*) must not be confused with Red Valerian (*Centranthus ruber* or *Valeriana ruber*), which should be taken only in very small doses and for only a day or two at a time. Valerian should be taken in moderation only, and for no more than a couple of weeks at a time.

ABOVE *Valerian is among the most diverse of herbs – one of its common names is "all heal."*

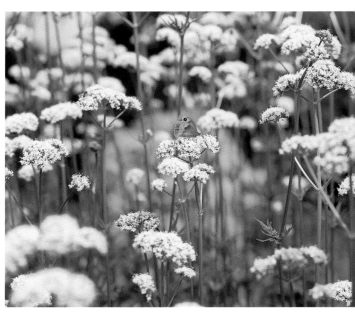

RIGHT *Valerian is crucial to the herbalist – its many valuable properties make it multi-purpose herb.*

Southernwood

This beautiful, feathery plant, one of many varieties of *Artemisia*, grows up to 4 ft. (1.2 m) high and is a soft gray-green color. This herb has many common names, all related to its association with courting: "lad's love," "old man," "maiden's ruin," and "kiss-in-my-corner." Southernwood's Latin name, *Artemisia,* was derived from the goddess Artemis (known as Diana to the Romans). Artemis was goddess of the hunt, nature, and also of the boundary between cultivation and the wilderness. She was also the moon goddess, so southernwood is associated with rituals involving the moon, or timed to coincide with the new moon.

Southernwood is sacred to the 5th century saint St. Ninian, whose feast day falls in the sign of Virgo, on September 16th. St. Ninian was Scottish, and southernwood was often used in Scotland to press between the pages of Bibles to perfume them.

ABOVE *Southernwood is a sacred herb associated with the sign of Virgo.*

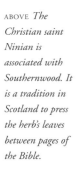

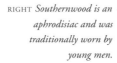

RIGHT *Southernwood is an aphrodisiac and was traditionally worn by young men.*

ABOVE *The Christian saint Ninian is associated with Southernwood. It is a tradition in Scotland to press the herb's leaves between pages of the Bible.*

LOVE POTION

Southernwood was believed to be an aphrodisiac and it was used to give (barely) coded love signals. A young man looking for a girl to woo would walk through the lanes sniffing a sprig of southernwood in his buttonhole. If any girl turned toward him as he passed, he would give her the sprig from his buttonhole. She would either reject him by throwing it on the ground, or she would smell it and then put her arm through his and they would walk together.

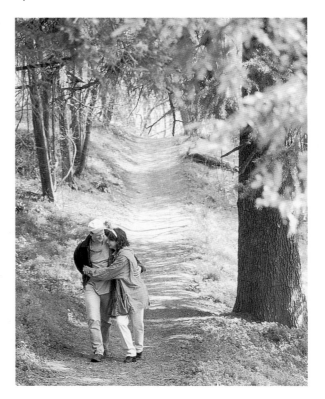

Healing with Southernwood

Southernwood tea makes a good tonic and helps to treat coughs and bronchial infections. A compress of southernwood is useful in treating cuts and grazes.

In traditional Chinese medicine, southernwood is also used to make moxibustion cones and sticks – these are lit and the sticks are left on the skin to create a deep warmth for treating rheumatism and aches and pains.

WARNING

Southernwood should not be taken during pregnancy.

Cooking with Southernwood

Southernwood is not generally used in cooking, although the leaves can be used in salads; be very sparing since the flavor is particularly strong.

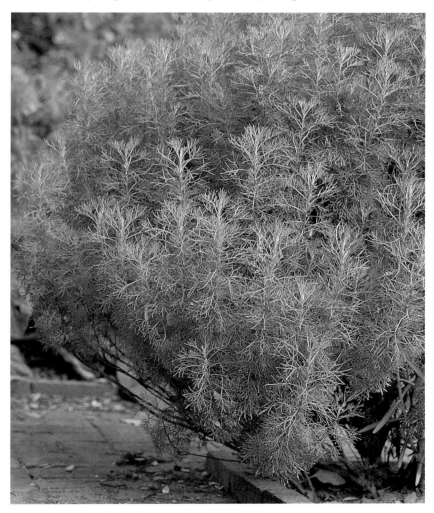

LEFT
Southernwood grows to quite a height, its feathery stems stretching upward as far as 4 ft.

Libra

SEPTEMBER 24 – OCTOBER 23

"These people are prodigal of their strengths and talents, and scatter their forces in all directions. They feel it their imperative duty to help everybody."

Eleanor Kirk *The Influence of the Zodiac upon Human Life*

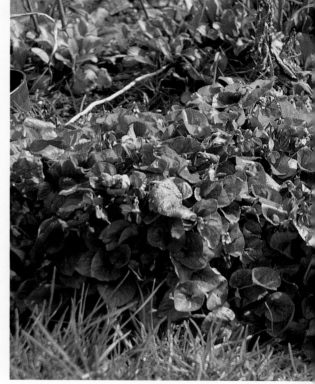

Libra, symbolized by the scales, is ruled by the planet Venus. The most important herbs linked to Libra are primrose, violet, and yarrow. Before exploring the qualities of these herbs, it is interesting to look at how the more seasonal herbs play a role in the traditional festivals and rituals held at this time of year.

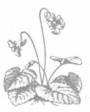

ABOVE *The violet is a Libran herb.*

Seasonal Rites

The most significant festival that falls within Libra is Michaelmas, the feast of St. Michael the Archangel, on September 29th. This marks the very end of the harvesting and is also the time when the autumn fairs and markets were held.

Michaelmas has always traditionally been a time of great feasting (especially on Michaelmas goose) and is also a very industrious period for pickling and preserving food to last the winter.

RIGHT *Violets, known as the garden pansy, are a colorful favorite of the gardener.*

Wild Blackberry

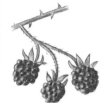

One of the most important herbs associated with this festival is the blackberry, which is usually at its best around this time. Its leaves are an important healing herb in the country, but at Michaelmas it is the berries that are gathered. They are full of the flavor of the rain and the sun and the earth which have nourished it through the summer, one of the most abundant of nature's wild fruits.

Traditionally, blackberries should not be harvested after Michaelmas, because after this date they are cursed by the devil. When he was cast out of heaven, so the legend tells, Satan landed in the middle of a bramble bush; this may be the reason for the ill will he reputedly bears toward the plant.

ABOVE *Wild blackberry has delicate blossoms before berries appear in early fall.*

LIBRA COMPLAINTS

Since the function of the kidneys is to maintain the balance of the body, it is appropriate that this part of the body should be governed by Libra, the scales. As it governs the kidneys, the sign rules complaints such as cystitis, kidney stones, enlarged prostate, and bedwetting in children. It does not necessarily follow that the Libra herbs are the most suitable herbs for treating problems related to this sign – for the best herbs to help cure Libra complaints, *see pages 124–27.*

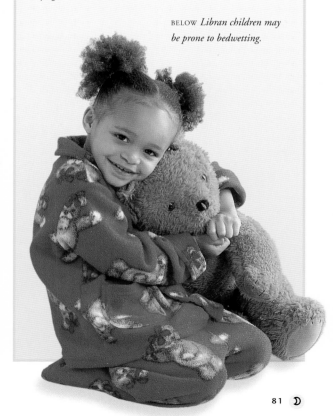

BELOW *Libran children may be prone to bedwetting.*

Violet

iolets are associated with modesty because they hide their flow-ers among their leaves. However, in some places, their dark color and the way they hang their heads made them a symbol of death and a bad omen. More often, though, they were considered a plant of humility in love.

Healing with Violet

Violet flowers can be taken in an infusion or a syrup as a mild laxative. They are also a sedative that will soothe headaches, anxiety, and insomnia, and they help coughs and bronchial complaints. The leaves or roots can be infused or decocted, and also help to ease colds, rhinitis, and bronchitis, and to soothe the effects of a hangover.

The most dramatic claims for violet as a healing herb are for the benefits of a poul-tice of the leaves. This has been used for thousands of years to cure skin cancers and is still used today as a gypsy remedy for tumors. An infusion of the leaves is said to cure some internal cancers. A poultice of the leaves is also used to soothe bruises, and sore, cracked nipples. For their decorative value, they can be crystallized and used as a garnish for desserts.

ABOVE Despite its small and pretty appearance, the violet has been associated with death – perhaps because the flower hangs downward.

HORSE CHARM

Violets also have a reputation for being able to calm horses, and were regularly worn as *boutonnières* at foxhunts, races, and horse sales.

Sweet violets were included, because of their scent, in the "drawing potions" that were used to calm the temperamental horses.

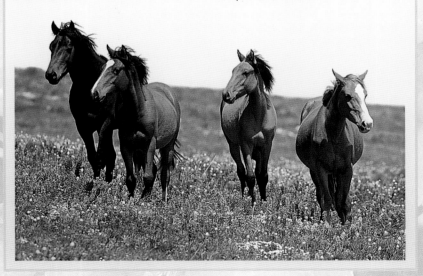

LEFT The modest violet is said to be powerful enough to subdue horses.

Cooking with Violet

Violet flowers, like those of primroses, are edible and can be added to salads in the spring. Sweet violet (*Viola odorata*) is more strongly flavored than others, but all types can be used. Violets are best known in cooking in their crystallized form, when they are used to decorate desserts, cakes, and ice cream.

CRYSTALLIZED VIOLETS

Primroses can also be crystallized in this way to make edible decorations.

1 EGG WHITE

SUPERFINE SUGAR

A HANDFUL OF VIOLET FLOWERS, STALKS REMOVED

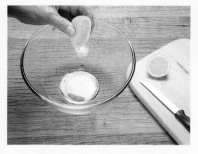

1 Lightly beat the egg white until it is just foaming. Place some superfine sugar in a small bowl. Place a sheet of waxed paper on a rack.

2 Dip a flower into the egg white, then dip it into the sugar to lightly coat. Place the flower on the sheet of waxed paper.

3 Repeat this process with the remaining flowers.

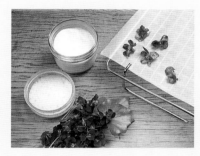

4 Cover the coated flowers with another sheet of waxed paper and dry them by putting them in a warm, dry place, such as or a very cool oven with the door open.

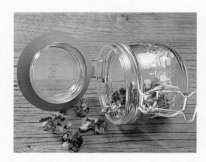

5 Once the flowers are dried, store in an airtight jar.

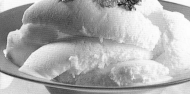

Primrose

This is a flower of shady woodland and hedge, which grows naturally in Europe. Its name means "first rose," and it is one of the earliest flowers of spring, sometimes even blooming in midwinter during mild spells.

Healing with Primrose

Primrose is a mild sedative, which is much less used now than it once was. You can use either the flowers or the whole plant to make an herbal tea that is a useful treatment for insomnia and anxiety. Primrose tea will help cure a headache, and it is also a mild cough remedy.

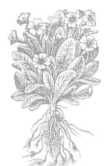

RIGHT *The primrose brightens hedges and shady banks in spring.*

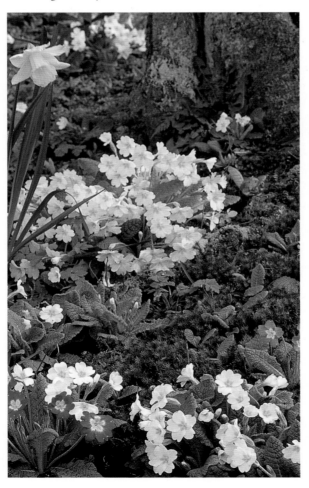

FAR RIGHT

Primroses can be made into an herbal tea to treat a cough.

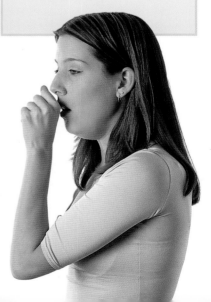

LOVE AND HOPE

Primroses are inextricably connected with spring, new life, young love, and bright hopes and pleasures. The expression "primrose path" means a path of pleasure. The phrase was first used by Shakespeare in Hamlet:

*Do not as some ungracious
  pastors do,
Show me the steep and thorny
  way to Heaven;
Whilst like a puffed and
  reckless libertine
Himself the primrose path
  of dalliance treads.*

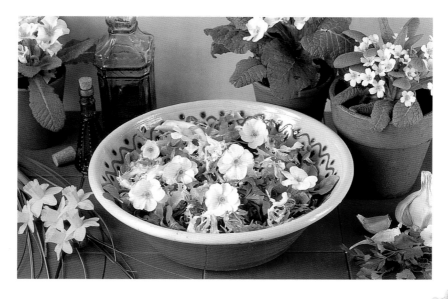

RIGHT *Edible
primrose flowers
make a pretty
addition to salad
dishes.*

Cooking with Primrose

Primrose makes a good culinary herb because the flowers, which are
edible, are so pretty. You can add the flowers to a green spring salad, or crystal-
lize them to use for decorating cakes and desserts. You can also cook primrose
leaves as a vegetable; boil or steam them, and serve them with a little butter.

MIXED LEAF AND PRIMROSE SALAD WITH
GRILLED GOAT'S CHEESE

*The leaves of the primrose are said to be ideal for salad; young tender
shoots can be cooked for greens or used in salads. While in bud, flower
stalks can also be eaten – raw or cooked.*

4 OZ (115G) MIXED DARK SALAD LEAVES
(ROCKET, SPINACH, AND LOLLO ROSSO)

2 OZ (55 G) WATERCRESS

2 OZ (55 G) YOUNG PRIMROSE LEAVES

8 OZ (225 G) CHERRY TOMATOES,
HALVED

1 TBSP OLIVE OIL

1 TBSP LEMON JUICE

9 OZ (250 G) GOAT'S CHEESE

1 Put the salad leaves, watercress, and
primrose leaves in a bowl and mix
together.

2 Preheat the grill to high. Cover a
rack with foil. Mix the lemon juice
and oil and drizzle over the goat's cheese.

3 Place on the rack and grill for 3 to 4
minutes until golden.

4 Top the salad with the cheese and
serve with a dressing of your choice.

ABOVE *The bright
yellow primrose
flowers are among
the first to decorate
hedges and verges
in the spring.*

Yarrow

Achilles was said to have cured his troops' wounds with yarrow, which is how it earned its Latin name, *Achillea millefolium*; the second part of the name means "thousand leaves" and refers to the featheriness of the plant. Yarrow has had a reputation for stemming the flow of blood since at least the time of the Greeks, and this explains many of its common names, including "staunch grass," "soldier's woundwort," "nosebleed," and "carpenter's weed" – this last one because it cures wounds inflicted by sharp tools like those carpenters use.

Healing with Yarrow

Yarrow has been used for centuries as a healing herb.

The most common use of yarrow is for stemming blood flow. A decoction or poultice of the leaves can be applied to wounds and rashes to help them heal, and an infusion helps to cure canker sores and sore gums.

FORETELLING THE FUTURE

Dried yarrow stalks were used for divination by the Druids, to prophecy the weather, and by the ancient Chinese, who used them in combination with the I Ching (The Book of Changes) to foretell the future.

ABOVE *Yarrow leaves are used to make a decoction or poultice to slow the flow of blood from wounds.*

RIGHT *The God Achilles was said to treat his own soldiers with yarrow; hence the plant's latin name,* Achillea millefolium.

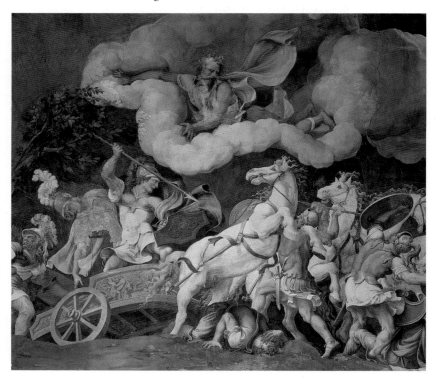

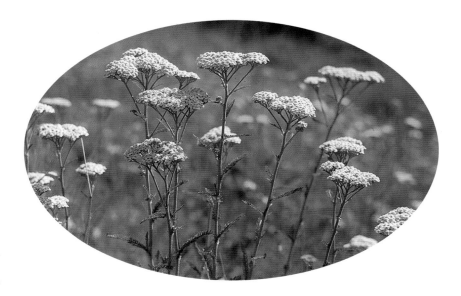

RIGHT *One of yarrow's traditional names is "thousand leaves" because of its feathery appearance.*

Yarrow tea is drunk to reduce menstrual flow, and it also induces sweats that help to cool fevers and cleanse the system. Fresh yarrow leaves can be chewed to ease toothache, and an ancient tradition suggests that the fresh leaves could be put into the nose to induce a nosebleed; the point of this was to ease the pain of a migraine. Yarrow tea also eases colds and flu, especially if you mix it with elderflowers and peppermint to create an all-round herbal cold treatment.

Yarrow was a traditional cure for consumption at one time, and has been used to treat dysentery and diarrhea. It also stimulates gastric secretion and in some places used to be given to cattle suffering from stomach complaints.

WARNING

Yarrow should be avoided in large doses or for prolonged periods because it can cause skin rashes, headaches, and vertigo. It should also be avoided during pregnancy.

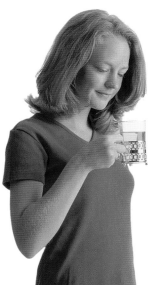

Cooking with Yarrow

Yarrow leaves taste peppery and slightly bitter, and can be used raw. Either use them in salads when they are still young and fresh, or chop them finely and add them to dips and cold sauces, or use them as a garnish.

LEFT *Yarrow tea is drunk to ease the symptoms of colds and flu.*

Scorpio

OCTOBER 24 – NOVEMBER 22

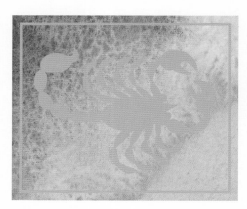

"THE SOLAR INFLUENCE PASSING THROUGH THIS SIGN WILL MAKE YOU A FIRM POWERFUL CHARACTER, ARISING FROM THE SILENT FORCE WITHIN, GIVING YOU ALSO OCCULT LEANINGS. YOU POSSESS MAGNETIC POWER, CRITICAL PERCEPTION AND ABILITY TO JUDGE KEENLY."

"SCORPIO" (WILLIAM F. ALLAN)
THE KEY TO YOUR OWN NATIVITY

$\mathcal{M}$ars is the traditional ruler of Scorpio and the key herbs of this sign are basil, tarragon, and wormwood. Before exploring the qualities of these herbs, it is interesting to take a look at the herbs that are in season during the Scorpio period, and discover how they play a part in rituals traditionally held at this time of year.

Seasonal Rites

The Celtic festival of Samhain, arguably the most important of all, is on October 31st. This coincides with the Christian festival of Hallowe'en or All Hallows Eve – the night before All Saints Day on November 1st. Samhain is the Celtic new year, and at midnight on October 31st it is time to say goodbye to the old, dying year and to greet the new.

As everyone knows, the crossover from one year to the next is the time when the veil between this world and the next is at its thinnest, and spirits are most likely to be seen. Many scrying (crystal-gazing) rituals were carried out on this night of the year, and many traditions tell of ways to see spirits, commune with those who have died, or divine the identity of a future husband or wife.

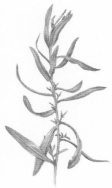

ABOVE *Tarragon is associated with the sun sign of Scorpio.*

BELOW *Hallowe'en falls in the Scorpio period. It is the night on which spirits are said to show themselves.*

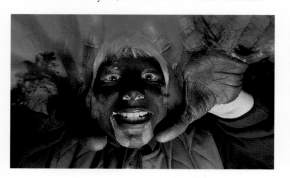

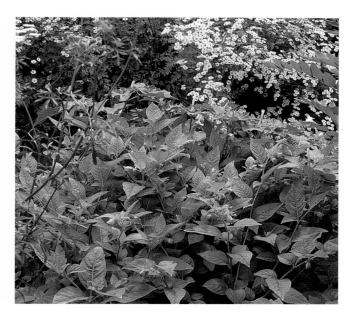

ABOVE *Deadly nightshade is an herb used in Samhain rituals. It is a poisonous hallucinogenic.*

The Samhain festival, like other Celtic rites, has always been centered around a bonfire, which keeps the new year alive and holds back evil spirits. Jack-o-lanterns were made from turnips or pumpkins and hung on gateposts on "Spunkie Night" for the same reason. This is the night when Herne the Hunter comes into his own, the unpredictable Green King who rules the winter time.

Samhain Herbs

Thyme is associated with death and rosemary with remembrance, so these two herbs are often incorporated into Samhain rituals. They commemorate both the old year and the souls of those who have died, and a sprig of one or other was traditionally worn on October 31st. Rue is also used in Samhain rituals, since it is the herb of repentance. When you enter the new year, it is wise to repent of all your ill deeds in the old year before you finally leave it behind you and move on.

Deadly nightshade is another plant associated with Samhain rites. Its Latin name, *Atropa belladonna*, derives from the Greek *Atropa*. Atropa was one of the three Fates, the one who cut the thread of human life. Many dark rituals include deadly nightshade, and it was one of the ingredients in witches' "flying ointment" – it seems that when this ointment was rubbed in, it produced a hallucinatory effect that made witches believe they were flying.

Deadly nightshade (which is very poisonous) was also taken in wine by the ancient Greek menads, who worshipped the god Dionysus, at their revels and orgies.

Dionysus was originally a pagan deity who became the god of wine and revelry, but he retained a wild, dangerous side much like the untamed aspect of Herne the Hunter.

RIGHT *Scorpios are ruled by Pluto and the very basic tenets of life: birth and death. For this reason they are prone to problems affecting libido.*

SCORPIO COMPLAINTS

Pluto, the planet ruling Scorpio, is associated with life, death, and renewal, so it is not surprising that this sign governs the genitals and the libido. Impotence, low libido, genito-urinary complaints – all these are the domain of Scorpio. It does not necessarily follow that the Scorpio herbs are the best herbs to treat these problems – for the most useful herbs to help Scorpio symptoms, *see pages 124–127.*

Basil

Basil was originally imported to Europe from the East. It has been cultivated in the Mediterranean for thousands of years, but only reached western Europe in the 16th century. Its name derives from a Greek phrase meaning "kingly herb," and basil is said to have sprung up around the tomb of Christ after the Resurrection.

In India, basil is considered sacred, so much so that it was chosen as the herb on which to swear oaths in court. It also grows on some Pacific islands, where it is sacred to the Haitian love goddess. In the West, however, it has been associated with the devil as much as with the divine.

In the past, the Greeks and Romans believed that basil would only grow if you uttered a curse as you sowed the seeds, and in the Middle Ages basil was associated with witchcraft.

Healing with Basil

Basil makes a useful tonic if you sniff the essential oil, or steep some of the leaves in wine for a few hours. Basil can be added to the bath in the form of an essential oil, or even as a bunch of fresh leaves, to help revive and invigorate.

A tea made from the leaves helps the digestion – or simply use the leaves in cooking to achieve the same effect. Basil is an especially popular herb added to Mediterranean cooking and is often used in vegetable-based recipes.

BELOW *Although we think of basil as a European herb, it was imported from the East and is sacred in India.*

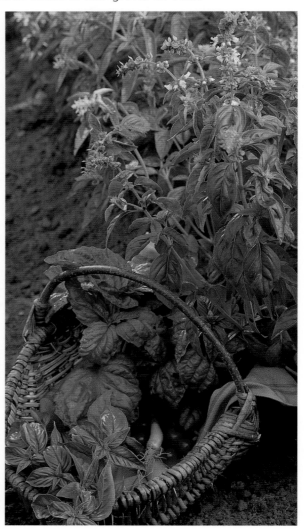

RIGHT *Many people expect to find basil in Mediterranean gardens.*

Cooking with Basil

Basil is an excellent culinary herb, which goes especially well with Mediterranean flavours such as garlic and tomatoes. The dried leaves taste of very little, so it is far better to use them fresh. Grow the plant in a pot on a warm sunny windowsill, or simply treat basil as a seasonal plant with a taste forever associated with summer.

There are many different varieties of basil, including purple-leafed basil, lemon basil, and cinnamon basil. Experiment with flavors to see which you prefer. The taste of basil doesn't combine particularly well with strong dark meat; use it instead with chicken, fish, eggs, cheese, and rice dishes. The leaves are better torn than chopped, or you can pound them with oil and use them in dressings and herb butter, or with French bread, or drizzled over salad or pizza.

Basil is the key ingredient in pesto sauce, along with pine kernels, garlic, Parmesan cheese, and oil. These are blended together into a sauce that is traditionally served with pasta and rice.

BELOW *The Cholmondeley sisters with their children (c.1600–1610). The Elizabethans believed that by holding a sprig of basil (along with a swallow's feather) a woman would not feel the pains of labor.*

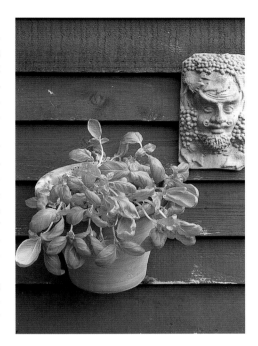

ABOVE *Basil likes sunny spots and is suitable for growing on patios, balconies, walls, and windowsills.*

WOMAN WISE

The Elizabethans held that if a woman in labor clutched a sprig of basil and a swallow's feather, she would feel no pain.

They also believed that a woman could not eat from a plate that had a sprig of basil hidden beneath it.

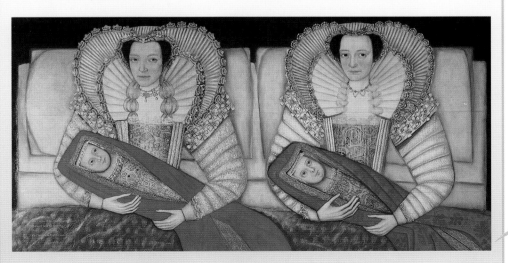

Tarragon

Yet another member of the *Artemisia* family (which has over 200 species), tarragon has long, narrow, pointed leaves. It grows to about 3 ft. (1m) tall and comes from southern Europe. In cooler climates it rarely flowers, so it needs to be propagated by cuttings or root division. Tarragon's Latin name is *Artemisia dranunculus; dranunculus* meaning little dragon, perhaps from the shape of the plant's roots. Certainly, having once acquired the name, tarragon was attributed with the power of healing snakebites and combating other poisons. There are two varieties of tarragon – the delicate French tarragon and the coarser Russian variety. Both are widely used, but the French variety is considered superior.

ABOVE *Dragon-like tarragon was once reputed to be an antidote to poison*

Healing with Tarragon

Tarragon is not widely used as a medicinal herb, but a tea made from it is a useful appetite stimulant and a general tonic for the digestive system. Tarragon used to be used as a cure for scurvy because it is high in vitamin C. Its leaves are also rich in vitamin A, iodine, and many mineral salts.

BELOW *Tarragon is not widely used as a medicinal herb, but it is a digestive tonic and a source of vitamin C.*

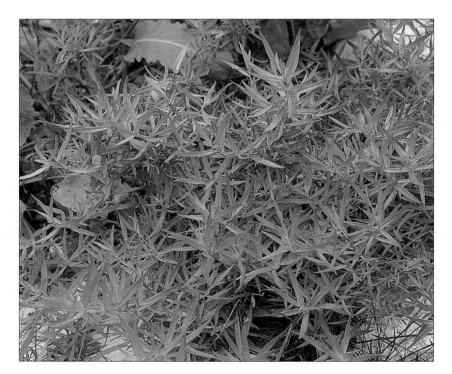

Cooking with Tarragon

Tarragon is a wonderful herb for cooking with, as long as you use it fresh. Its flavor complements chicken and fish particularly, and goes well in salads and egg dishes. It is one of the standard ingredients of *fines herbes*, and it is excellent in cream sauces, soups, salad dressings, and stuffings for fish.

Try chopping tarragon finely and using it in stuffed tomatoes, rice dishes such as cold rice salads, in mayonnaise to accompany fish such as salmon, and in herb butter to cook with vegetables or broiled meat.

Tarragon is one of the key ingredients in béarnaise sauce, a classic warm sauce traditionally served with broiled meat and fish.

BÉARNAISE SAUCE

1 TSP. TARRAGON VINEGAR

½ OZ. (15G) CHOPPED SHALLOTS

6 CRUSHED PEPPERCORNS

¼ OZ. (5G) TARRAGON SPRIGS

3 EGG YOLKS

8 OZ. (225G) WARM, MELTED BUTTER

1 SPRIG OF FINELY CHOPPED CHERVIL

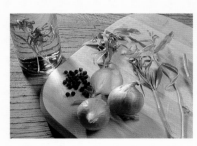

1 Put the vinegar, shallots, peppercorns, and stalks of tarragon in a small boiler and reduce. Add a tablespoon of cold water and leave to cool.

2 Add the egg yolks and whisk well. Return to a low heat and whisk until you have a sabayon – a cream thick enough to stand up. Do not overheat the yolks.

3 Remove the pan from the heat and allow the sabayon to cool a little.

4 Gradually whisk in the warm, melted butter, whisking well after each addition to ensure it is fully combined before you add any more.

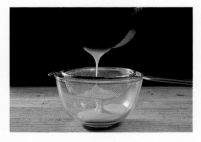

5 Strain the sauce through muslin or a very fine sieve.

6 Finely chop the tarragon leaves and add to the sauce with the chervil. Serve warm.

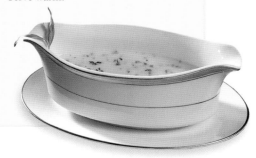

Wormwood

Wormwood is another *artemisia – Artemisia absinthium*. The second part of the Latin name for this plant, *Absinthium*, comes from the Latin for "desist from," so the entire name means to desist from Artemis. Since Artemis was a virgin goddess, presumably this was good advice. Wormwood was said to flourish in the path of the serpent in the Garden of Eden, which supposedly explains why its taste is so bitter. It was included in the manufacture of ink because the flavor deterred mice from eating old letters. Wormwood was commonly used as an insecticide, as a strewing herb, and hung up among clothes or in the granary to deter rats and mice. A weak decoction can be used as an insecticidal spray, but don't spray it on other plants.

Wormwood was used to flavor aperitifs including absinthe and vermouth, the former of which derives its name from the Latin name for the plant. The English name wormwood (and the French vermouth) is a corruption of the German herb wine named wermut. It is not a culinary herb.

Healing with Wormwood

Wormwood, curiously enough, is useful for expelling worms even though this isn't how it got its name. It is particularly effective against roundworms and threadworms. Like tarragon, it also works on the digestive system, stimulating the appetite and the digestive juices, and it acts as a tonic for the liver and gall bladder.

Wormwood also used to function as a prompt to bring on menstruation. It takes its Latin name from the goddess Artemis, who protected women in childbirth, and it was a popular women's herb. It was applied as a compress to speed up labor and taken afterward to help expel the afterbirth.

ABOVE *The healing properties of wormwood are indicated by its name; it is used to treat roundworm and threadworm.*

LEFT *Wormwood is used to flavor aperitifs such as absinthe.*

Wormwood as an antiseptic

Wormwood is traditionally used in a vinegar known as "Four Thieves." It is not used internally, but as an antiseptic rub or kitchen cleaner. It can also be added to your bath for a refreshing and cleansing soak.

The origin of the name "Four Thieves" is rather sinister: it comes from the practice of robbers rubbing the concoction all over their bodies to protect themselves before plundering the corpses of plague victims. This would have been common practice across Europe in the late Middle Ages and during the Renaissance when the plague was especially rife.

Four Thieves vinegar is made by adding a tablespoon of each of the following fresh chopped herbs: wormwood, lavender, rosemary, and sage to 2 pints (1 liter) of vinegar. Use this combination fresh, or strain the mixture before bottling it.

SAFETY CHARM

Wormwood is claimed to protect against evil and ill-fortune, and was often hung by the door to keep the house safe. To this day, Italian drivers sometimes still tie bunches of wormwood to the stem of the rearview mirror to protect them on steep mountain roads.

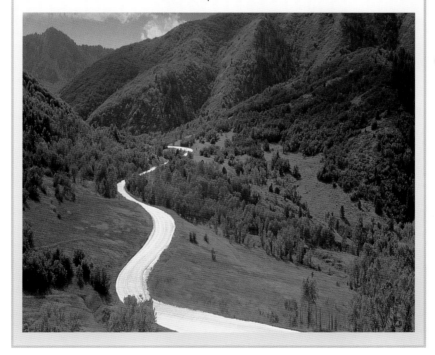

ABOVE *Wormwood should be avoided during pregnancy.*

RIGHT *Some drivers protect themselves on mountainous roads with a stem of wormwood.*

Sagittarius

NOVEMBER 23 – DECEMBER 21

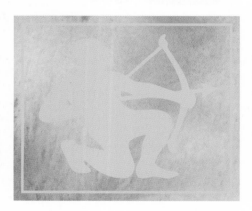

"THOSE BELONGING TO SAGITTARIUS ARE BOLD, ZEALOUS, DETERMINED AND COMBATIVE. VERY QUICK TO DECIDE, ACT AND SPEAK, THEIR MIND IS CONSTANTLY RUNNING AHEAD. GOING BEYOND THE PRESENT, THEY HAVE A TENDENCY TO PEER INTO THE FUTURE, AND TO FORESEE EVENTS."

"SEPHARIEL" (WALTER GORN OLD)
THE ASTROLOGERS' MAGAZINE NO. 34

The herbs associated with Sagittarius, through the influence of the ruling planet Jupiter, are sage, mallow, and feverfew. Before we explore the properties of these herbs, it is interesting to look at the way the seasonal herbs of the Sagittarius period play a role in the festivals and rituals traditionally held at this time of year.

Seasonal Rites

Yule, the Celtic festival to celebrate the winter solstice, usually falls on December 21st, the shortest day of the year (occasionally the shortest day is the 22nd). This is the time when the winter is at its darkest, although the coldest time is still to come. So the Yule festival is a reminder that even though the world looks dead, it is not.

Holly and ivy are used as decorations because they are among the few evergreen plants that symbolize life and reassure us that spring will eventually return.

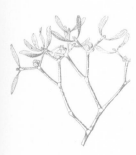

ABOVE *Mistletoe is an herb for midwinter, revered particularly by the Celts.*

MYSTICAL MISTLETOE

The mistletoe was the sacred plant of the Celts. It grew on their revered oak trees (as well as other trees), and it was believed that the berries contained the semen of the oak god or spirit. The Druids collected mistletoe with great ceremony. It was cut with a golden knife on a particular day of the lunar cycle and was caught in a white cloth before it reached the ground.

Mistletoe was thought to be an exceedingly powerful plant, with formidable healing properties. It also protected against witchcraft and lightning, and had the power to promote fertility. At Yule, it has always been thought unlucky to leave mistletoe out of the decorations, and it is a common ritual to keep each year's mistletoe until the following year, when it should be burned beneath the Yule log.

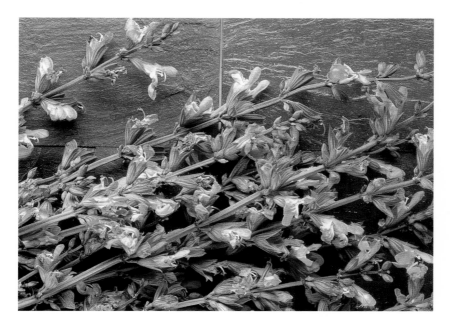

LEFT *Sage has small tubular lilac flowers in June and July, but is associated with the sun sign of Sagittarius.*

Evergreens are also the sanctuary for the spirits of other plants, whose own natural homes offer no refuge at this time of year. So by bringing branches of holly and ivy indoors, people have traditionally offered shelter to the nature spirits.

The Yule log should traditionally be found, rather than bought, and must not be brought into the house until the day itself. It must be lit ceremonially from a fragment of the previous year's Yule log and must burn all night. Ideally, the log – or at least the fire – should not go out for twelve days, so that the fire of life still burns through the darkest part of winter. And of course, a piece must be saved for next year.

The Sagittarius herb sage is an evergreen and is therefore another important winter plant, reminding us that the dark days will not last forever. Its pungent aroma led it to be used as an incense in rituals.

RIGHT *It is traditional to hang an evergreen wreath on your door as part of the Christmas festivities.*

SAGITTARIUS COMPLAINTS

Jupiter, the traditional ruler of Sagittarius, is concerned with learning and philosophy, and also with travel; Jupiter has a tendency to excess, and is therefore associated with the liver. The sign therefore governs illnesses and diseases of this part of the body. The Sagittarius herbs may not necessarily be the right herbs to cure these problems – for the herbs most suitable for treating Sagittarius symptoms, *see pages 124–127.*

Sage

There are over 750 varieties of sage worldwide, but the most important herb is *Salvia officinalis*. It has always been considered a healing herb, and the name comes from the Latin *salveo* meaning "I heal." It was long thought that sage had such powers that it could render you virtually immortal; the Chinese have a saying "How can a man grow old if he grows sage in his garden?" The Chinese valued sage tea so highly that they used to exchange their local tea with the Dutch for sage tea, bartering it weight for weight.

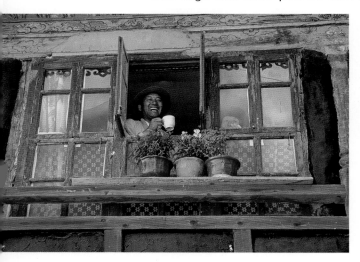

The Romans regarded sage as a sacred herb and harvested it with great ceremony. They cleansed and purified themselves thoroughly, made sacrifices of food, and cut the sage with a special ceremonial knife.

ABOVE *Over 750 varieties of sage grow across the world.*

Healing with Sage

ABOVE *Sage is a particularly useful herb for women. Fresh sage leaves can be eaten or made into an infusion.*

Sage is indeed, as people have recognized for centuries, an incredibly valuable medicinal herb with a wide range of healing properties. Sage tea is particularly good for the liver and the digestion.

Sage tea also helps against diarrhea and is an excellent tonic for the nervous system as well as for the blood. It contains the hormone estrogen and is used often used to treat menopause or irregular menstruation in women.

The leaf, eaten fresh or drunk as an infusion, is excellent to combat colds, sore throats, coughs, and laryngitis. Sage also eases infections of the mouth, such as ulcers and inflamed gums. It helps to reduce sweating and bring down a fever.

WARNING

Sage should not be taken in large amounts for extended periods, since its antiseptic properties can become toxic in their effect.

WOMEN RULE

Sage is one of the herbs which is said to flourish in the gardens of households ruled by the woman, and where the sage thrives, the woman shall bear all daughters and no sons. Many traditional folk rhymes confirm this, such as:

If the sage bush thrives and grows
The master's not master...
and he knows.

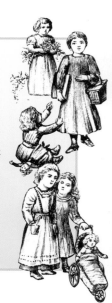

Cooking with Sage

Sage is one of the staple culinary herbs, all the more useful because it is evergreen and can be used fresh all year round. It has a strong flavor, so err on the side of caution or you could overdo the taste. But it is worth incorporating into much of your cooking, since its flavor is excellent, especially with fatty meat; it helps the body to digest greasy food, so it is a healthy as well as a tasty combination. It is an herb that can be used well with either sweet or nonsweet dishes.

One of the classic sage combinations is with onion, and sage and onion dressing is wonderful for poultry dressing – not only chicken, but also turkey, duck, or goose. Sage also goes well with pork and is ideal to use in homemade sausages. It also complements the taste of liver and can be added to liver and bacon gravy for a classic traditional dish.

Sage butter can be served with broiled meat, particularly lamb, steak, venison, and other strong meat, and sage oil is wonderful as a base for frying onions for stews.

Among the sweet dishes, the flavor of sage goes best with orange. You can make an excellent sugar syrup flavored with sage to pour over peeled oranges.

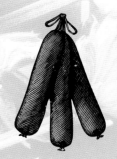

ABOVE *Sage is a popular herb to add to meat, especially sausages.*

SAGE AND ONION STUFFING

2 OZ. (50G) BUTTER OR LARD

2 OZ. (50G) CHOPPED ONION

4 OZ. (100G) WHITE BREAD CRUMBS

1 TBL CHOPPED SAGE

PINCH OF CHOPPED PARSLEY

SALT AND PEPPER

1 Heat the fat in a skillet, add the onion, and cook until soft but not browned.

2 Add the rest of the ingredients and stir to combine.

3 Use to stuff poultry or a pork joint, and roast as required.

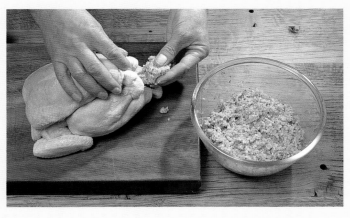

Mallow

Mallow's edible seedheads are a curious shape and have given rise to many of its common names – "billy buttons," "pancake," "cheese flower," and "biscuits." The Latin word malva, meaning soft, gave mallow its Latin name (*Malva sylvestris*), from which its common name derives. The Greeks and Romans used it medicinally and ate it as a vegetable.

Musk mallow *(Malva moschata)* has similar properties to common mallow, and some people prefer its flavor in cooking. Its name derives from the musky smell of the crushed leaves. Marshmallow *(Althaea officinalis)* is often preferred for medicinal uses. It is more potent than the other mallows; its name comes from the Latin *altheo*, meaning "I cure."

BELOW *Mallow as a decoction or infusion makes a good antiseptic mouthwash.*

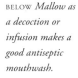

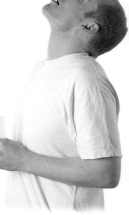

ANTIDOTE TO LOVE

In the Middle Ages one of the most popular uses for mallow was as an antidote to protect against love potions, because of its supposedly sedative properties.

The idea was to dull the senses so as to make one unreceptive to love charms.

Healing with Mallow

Mallow is used to treat skin complaints such as cuts, rashes, ulcers, boils, and wounds. Either make a compress, or add a decoction to the bath water to ease extensive skin rashes. A mouthwash or gargle with a decoction or infusion will help to soothe inflamed gums and canker sores.

An infusion of mallow acts as a mild laxative and is helpful for soothing gastrointestinal complaints. It is also useful in treating chest infections including coughs, bronchitis, and other irritating complaints.

BELOW *Mallow is commonly used as a decoction to ease skin disorders.*

Cooking with Mallow

Mallow leaves can be eaten in salads or cooked as a vegetable; try steaming them or lightly boiling them, much as you would spinach. The seeds and seedpods can be eaten in salads; they used to be picked and eaten straight from the plant as a delicacy, in the way we pick and eat blackberries nowadays.

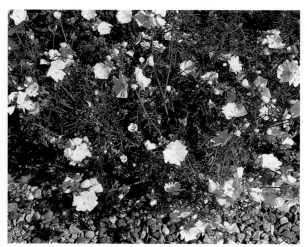

RIGHT *The mallow is a popular garden flower, blooming throughout the summer mouths.*

Feverfew

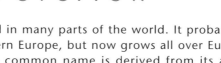

This herb grows wild in many parts of the world. It probably originated in southeastern Europe, but now grows all over Europe and North America. Its common name is derived from its ability to reduce fevers, and Culpeper recommended it in his 17th century herbal for headaches and colds. Feverfew was also used to treat melancholy. By the late 18th century it was considered valuable for treating people who were suffering from an excess of opium.

Healing with Feverfew

Feverfew has long been recognized – although not that widely used – as a cure for headaches. Recently, however, research has shown that it is highly effective for treating headaches and migraines, especially if taken every day as a preventative by chronic sufferers. The trials were particularly impressive because feverfew performed better than the most effective drug on the market. Feverfew leaves are very bitter, and the best way to take them is to put three or four leaves in a sandwich. Eaten every day, this reduces or cures migraines in the majority of people.

The trials that were conducted into feverfew threw up other unexpected results. Almost half of those people tested reported other improvements in their health as a result of taking feverfew. These included better sleep and reduced pain from arthritis. Fewer than one in five people reported unpleasant side effects, mostly canker sores or numbness of the tongue. These side effects can sometimes be avoided by taking the herb in tablet form.

BELOW *The feverfew flower looks a little like a daisy and grows wild across Europe and North America.*

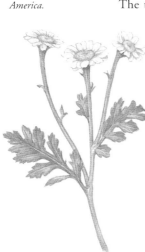

ABOVE *Feverfew flourishes in this bed and serves as a backdrop to pink poppies.*

Cooking with Feverfew

Feverfew is a very bitter herb, and despite its use as a treatment for stomach disorders is not recommended for culinary purposes.

Capricorn

DECEMBER 22 – JANUARY 20

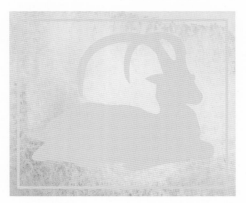

"A FRIEND ONCE IS A FRIEND ALWAYS. THEY ARE USUALLY CAREFUL IN ALL MONEY AND BUSINESS AFFAIRS, AND A PROMISE IS SACREDLY REGARDED. THEY ARE NATURAL PLANNERS, AND KNOW HOW TO MAKE BOTH ENDS MEET."

ELEANOR KIRK, THE INFLUENCE OF THE ZODIAC UPON HUMAN LIFE

The ruling planet of Capricorn, the astrological sign of midwinter, is Saturn, and the herbs that come under this sign are sorrel, Solomon's seal, and comfrey. Before we explore the particular qualities of these herbs, it is interesting to look at how seasonal herbs play a role in the traditional festivals and rituals that fall within Capricorn.

Seasonal Rites

The Celtic festival of Yule occasionally falls within Capricorn rather than Sagittarius, but the more recently established Christmas festival always does, as do the twelve days following, which are traditionally a time of feasting and celebration.

Christmas Rose

One of the herbal plants most closely associated with this time of year is the black hellebore (*Helleborus niger*) which is, perversely, white (it is named after its black root). This beautiful flower is also known as the Christmas Rose because it is often in flower on Christmas Day, December 25th. Its ability to flower even in the middle of winter has earned it a reputation as a magical herb.

The Christmas Rose is a sacred plant of protection and should be introduced into the house on Christmas Day to bring blessing to all the family. Do not cut the flowers, however, but keep the plant in a pot to transport it indoors.

ABOVE *Solomon's seal is associated with the astrological sign of Capricorn.*

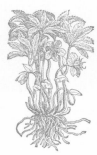

ABOVE *The* Helleborus niger, *or Christmas Rose, has leathery dark green leaves and white flowers.*

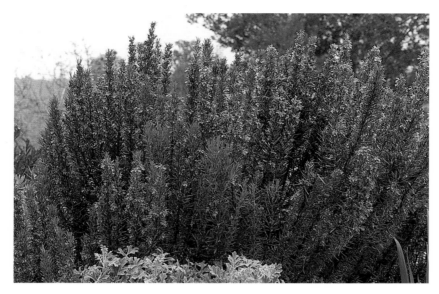

RIGHT *Rosemary is considered a holy herb; the blue flowers are said to have been colored by the Virgin Mary's cloak.*

Holy Herb

Another Christmas herb is rosemary, which is a holy herb. The story is that the flowers were once white, but on her flight into Egypt, the Virgin Mary spread out her blue cloak to dry on a rosemary bush and the flowers turned blue; they have been blue ever since. Rosemary is said to flower at midnight on Christmas Eve. A sprig of rosemary, preferably in flower, should always feature somewhere in the Christmas decorations.

Saturnalia

Another ancient festival that falls at this time, ending on December 25th, is the Roman Saturnalia (Capricorn is ruled by Saturn). During this festival, masters and servants changed roles; to this day the officers of the British army wait on their men and serve Christmas dinner. The Catholic Church outlawed Saturnalia, but it left its legacy, including a custom by which one servant was crowned Lord of Misrule and allowed to preside over the Christmas household with wild revelry.

The herb most strongly identified with Saturnalia is bay (*Laurus nobilis*), which is sacred to the god of medicine, Apollo. Bay is a strong herb of protection and was used by the ancients against evil, lightning, illness, and disease. It is evergreen and was therefore considered at its most powerful during winter when other herbs were not to be found. A bay tree planted beside the front door is a symbol of protection for the household.

CAPRICORN COMPLAINTS

Saturn, the ruling planet of Capricorn, represents order and limitation. The physical body is ordered, its movement limited by its bones and joints – it follows that these parts of the body are the domain of Capricorn. The sign of Capricorn therefore governs diseases such as arthritis, osteoporosis, and backache. However, the herbs belonging to this sign may not necessarily be the best herbs to treat these problems – for the most suitable herbs to help Capricorn symptoms, *see pages 124–127.*

RIGHT *Those born under the sun-sign of Capricorn are likely to suffer from backache.*

Sorrel

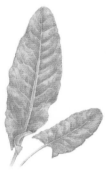

Sorrel is native to Europe and Asia, and naturalized in North America. It has a sharp taste, and the leaves were often sucked to relieve thirst and even – according to some – to cure spots. Children used to suck the stems or chew the leaves and spit them out after extracting the sour juice. The Latin name *Rumex* comes from the Latin word meaning "to suck"; the common name "sorrel" comes from the old French word for sour: *surelle*.

This practice of sucking or chewing sorrel leaves gave rise to numerous folk names for sorrel, such as sour dock, sour sabs, sour grabs, sour leeks, and sour grass – all a good indication of its flavor.

There are two main varieties of sorrel: common or garden sorrel, *Rumex acetosa*; and French sorrel, *Rumex scutatus*, also known as Buckler leaf sorrel. French sorrel has smaller leaves and is less acidic, and is generally considered superior.

ABOVE *Sorrel leaves are said to relieve thirst if sucked.*

SORREL SOUFFLÉ

you will need:

5 TBL. (60G) BUTTER

3 CUPS (25G) FRESH YOUNG SORREL LEAVES

3 TBL. (40G) ALL-PURPOSE FLOUR

1¼ CUPS (300 ML) MILK

5 EGGS SEPARATED

2 TBL. (40G) GRATED PARMESAN CHEESE

SALT AND PEPPER TO SEASON

1 Melt 1 TBL. oz (15g) of butter in a large saucepan and add the sorrel. Cook over a moderate heat until tender, about 6 or 7 minutes. Drain and squeeze, then chop. Keep back enough butter to grease the soufflé dish, and melt the rest. Stir in the flour. Slowly add the milk a little at time, stirring thoroughly to prevent lumps, to make a white sauce.

2 Leave the sauce to cool a little, then add four of the egg yolks. Add the sorrel, parmesan, and seasoning and stir until well mixed.

3 Prepare a 3-pint (1½-liter) soufflé dish by buttering it and tying a piece of buttered parchment paper around it; the paper should stand 2 in. (5 cm) above the rim of the dish. Preheat the oven to 200°C/400°F/ Gas mark 6.

4 In a clean bowl, whisk the five egg whites until they are stiff. Stir 2 TBL. of egg white into the soufflé mixture already prepared, and then fold in the rest with a metal spoon.

5 Pour the mixture into the soufflé dish and put it in the preheated oven. Bake for about 25 minutes until risen and golden on top. Serve immediately.

Healing with Sorrel

Sorrel leaves can be infused and drunk as a tea to treat liver and kidney complaints. It also makes a useful gargle or mouth wash for mouth ulcers, or a wash for infected cuts and boils.

You can make a poultice of the leaves and apply it to skin conditions such as spots and acne; the juice will help to heal the skin.

Cooking with Sorrel

Sorrel leaves were once used widely in cooking, but are now largely neglected. Sorrel is similar to spinach and can be cooked the same way, although its flavor is more acid. Sorrel is not widely available in grocery stores and supermarkets, but good restaurants know better than to ignore this herb, and many use it effectively in many dishes. It is much more common in France and the Mediterranean.

Sorrel can be eaten raw and is an ideal constituent in green salads, although it's wise to use a slightly sweet dressing to offset the natural sharpness. If you boil sorrel in water in the same way you might cook spinach, change the water halfway through the cooking to remove some of the acidity.

The flavor of sorrel goes very well with poultry, fish, and eggs. You can add finely chopped sorrel to omelets and quiches, and use it in sauces for fish and meat. Because sorrel has such an acid taste, it is generally either used in small quantities or combined with another vegetable to take the edge off the sharpness. Use vegetables that cook at the same speed and in the same way so you can prepare and cook them all together. Lettuce, spinach, or watercress go particularly well with sorrel.

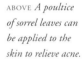

ABOVE *A poultice of sorrel leaves can be applied to the skin to relieve acne.*

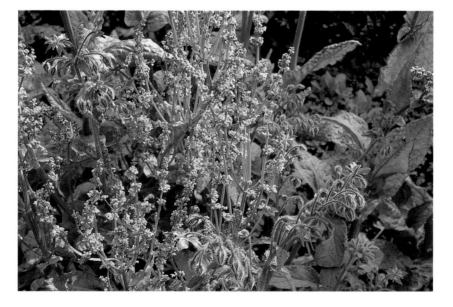

RIGHT *Sorrel can be grown among flowers in beds and picked fresh to add to salads and sauces.*

SORREL AND WATERCRESS SOUP

4 OZ. (100G) SORREL

4 OZ. (100G) WATERCRESS

2 OZ. (50G) BUTTER

4 OZ. (100G) PEELED AND CUBED
POTATOES

2½ CUPS (600ML) CHICKEN BROTH

¾ cup (150ML) LIGHT CREAM

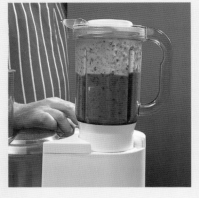

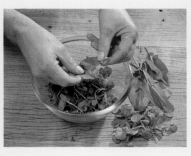

1 Wash the sorrel and watercress, dry
them, and tear into small pieces.

2 Melt the butter in a skillet and add
the sorrel and watercress. Stew the
vegetables over a low heat for about 5
minutes, until well cooked.

3 Add the potatoes and broth and
bring to a boil. Cover and simmer
for about 25 minutes.

4 Remove from the heat and let it
cool a little, then purée the soup.

5 Return the soup to the pan and
heat it without quite bringing to a
boil. Add the cream and serve
immediately.

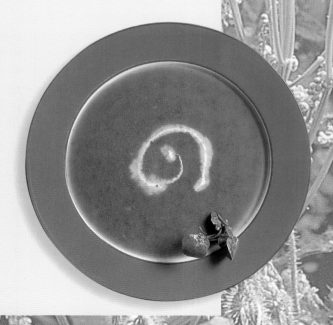

Solomon's Seal

The first part of the Latin name for this plant, *Polygonatum biflorum,* comes from the Greek words meaning "many knees," because the rhizome has many bulbous, lumpy joints. The common name is said to come from the fact that King Solomon himself put the seal of approval on using the plant's roots as a medicine. An alternative explanation is that the marks on the roots resemble Hebrew seals.

Solomon's seal has many common names, most of which refer in some way to its appearance: "drop berry," "lady's lockets," "ladder to heaven," "David's harp," and "Jacob's ladder" (a particularly confusing name, since it is also used – and more often – to describe a completely different plant).

ABOVE *King Solomon is said to have approved the use of the herb* Polygonatum biflorum, *giving it its common name – Solomon's Seal.*

WARNING

All parts of Solomon's seal are poisonous, and should be taken only under strict medical supervision.

Healing with Solomon's Seal

Solomon's seal rhizomes can be used to make an effective poultice for reducing the inflammation surrounding sprains and broken bones.

The rhizomes are also helpful for treating skin problems, wounds, and bruises, and they are said to remove the color from a black eye. Native Americans made a tea from the roots which they used to treat menstrual problems and internal discomfort. The Chinese use the plant in their traditional medicine as a treatment for diabetes, since one of its active ingredients lowers blood sugar levels.

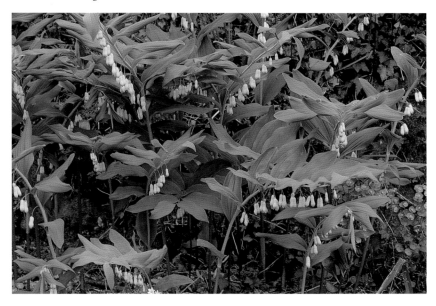

RIGHT *The Native North Americans recognized the herbal value of Solomon's seal and used it to treat menstrual disorders and internal problems.*

Comfrey

Comfrey grows naturally in parts of Europe and Asia, and was probably distributed through large parts of the rest of Europe by the Crusaders, who called it "Saracen's root," having seen the enemy use it to heal injuries. Comfrey roots were pulped into a mucilaginous mass and laid on pieces of leather, which were then wrapped around broken limbs (a condition very much associated with the Capricorn sign). The pounded root, once dried out, would set rigid like plaster and hold the bones in place while they healed. This gave rise to other common names such as "knitbone," "boneset," and "knitback."

ABOVE *Comfrey will grow in most habitats and its bell-shaped flowers change from an initial pink to bright blue.*

AMAZING POWERS

Comfrey has many other healing properties and was credited with such healing powers that one country belief was that comfrey leaves added to the bathwater would restore virginity.

FIRST AID TIP

A tube of purchased comfrey cream is a useful item to keep in a first-aid box, good for helping the healing process on bruises, sprains, and minor fractures. (Not for use on broken skin.)

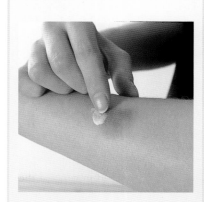

ABOVE *Comfrey is an extremely potent healer and is ideal to treat wounds of many kinds.*

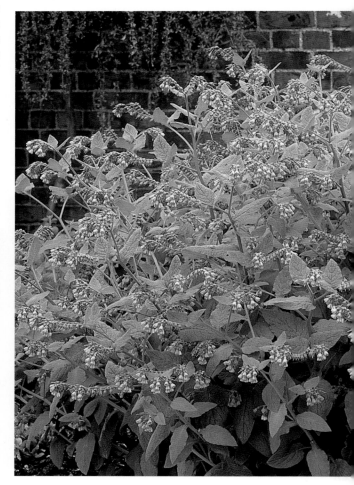

Healing with Comfrey

Comfrey is a valuable healing herb, not only for its ability to set like plaster (which is arguably not needed these days), but also because it heals the Capricorn conditions of aching and arthritic joints and muscle sprains. It can also help with diseases of the bone such as osteoporosis.

There are several ways of treating these conditions using comfrey; you can spread bruised leaves directly on the affected area or, for more serious conditions, you can make a poultice of the leaf or root; the other option is to wash the area regularly with an infusion or decoction of comfrey.

A multi-purpose remedy can be made by packing a quantity of comfrey leaves into an airtight jar and leaving it in a dark place for about two years. You will find that the leaves have produced a golden oil which, when strained, can be used to rub into sores, ulcers, and arthritic joints.

The above treatment is also excellent for relief from the following: ulcers, burns, varicose veins, and eczema.

One of comfrey's other potentially valuable constituents is protein. Some varieties consist of nearly 35 percent pure protein, which is as high a level as soybeans. Commercial attempts to extract the protein – along the same lines as soybeans – have so far failed, but it means that comfrey has a strong nutritional value when eaten as a vegetable. It also contains many other minerals and vitamins, including vitamin B12.

Cooking with Comfrey

Comfrey is rarely used in cooking these days, but used to be popular across Europe. You can eat the new leaves raw in salads or cooked rather like spinach, or even made into a mousse. The stems can be blanched much as you treat asparagus.

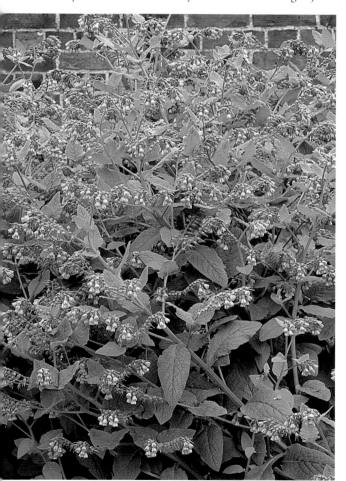

BELOW Comfrey has delicate mauve flowers. The Crusaders were responsible for bringing comfrey – which they called "Saracen's root" – to Europe.

NATURAL FERTILIZER

Comfrey has also been widely used for centuries as a natural, organic liquid fertilizer, since it has an exceptionally high potassium content. Soak the leaves in water for about four weeks, and then use the liquid to feed tomatoes, potatoes, beans, and other fruit and vegetables that need potash.

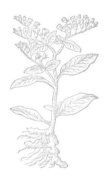

ABOVE Comfrey is a rich source of protein and vitamin B$_{12}$, and its leaves can be cooked and eaten much the same as spinach leaves.

Aquarius

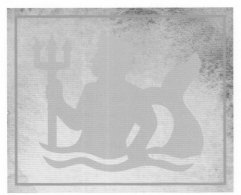

JANUARY 21 – FEBRUARY 19

"The chief characteristic of the typical Aquarian is.... his extraordinary breadth of vision. He is absolutely unbiased and open-minded, without taint of prejudice or superstition of any kind. Tradition and authority leave him untouched."

Isabelle M. Pagan *From Pioneer to Poet*

Uranus is the ruling planet of Aquarius, and the key herbs of this sign are elder, fumitory, and mullein. Before we explore the qualities of these herbs, it is interesting to look at how the more seasonal herbs of the Aquarius cycle play a role in the traditional festivals and rituals held at this time of the year.

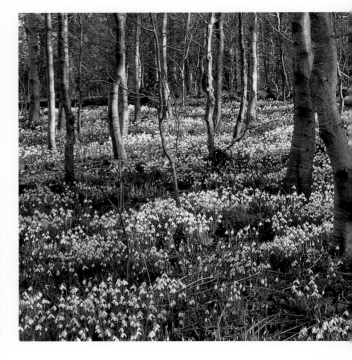

UNLUCKY SNOWDROPS

Snowdrops are seen by some as unlucky, and many people will not have them in the house. However, others view them as a sacred herb. White is the color of purity, and the way that snowdrops hang their heads is a symbol of modesty; for this reason they also represent virginity. Their common names include "fair maids of February," "Christ's flower," "the purification flower," and "Candlemas bells."

Seasonal Rites

The Celtic festival of Imbolc falls on February 2nd, celebrating the first stirrings of spring and the start of the lambing season. It is a peaceful and joyful celebration, and the ritual of welcoming the spring is decorated with early spring herbs and flowers such as primroses and, especially, snowdrops since the ritual color for Imbolc is white.

The Christian counterpart to Imbolc is Candlemas, the feast of the Purification of the Virgin Mary. This festival is a celebration of child-bearing, and one of the herbs commonly associated with it is box. At this time of year, box takes over from holly and ivy as the evergreen ritual plant; it is a strong protective plant and was traditionally grown to protect against both witches and the plague. Box is commonly used to create hedges, especially for mazes.

BELOW *The festival of Imbolc is celebrated early in the year and associated with flowers such as snowdrops, shown here dominating a woodland.*

AQUARIUS COMPLAINTS

Uranus, the ruling planet of Aquarius, represents the individual. Anyone who knows an Aquarian well will recognize the individuality of people born under this sign. Since the whole person or individual is enclosed within the skin – the outer appearance of the person – so it is the skin and all its conditions that Aquarius governs. Consequently, typical Aquarian complaints include acne, spots, boils, psoriasis and eczema. It does not necessarily follow that the Aquarius herbs are the best remedies to treat these problems – for the most useful herbs to help Aquarius symptoms, *see pages 124–127.*

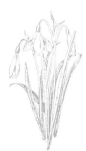

ABOVE *Snowdrops are among the first brave plants to break through the earth in springtime, under the sign of Aquarius.*

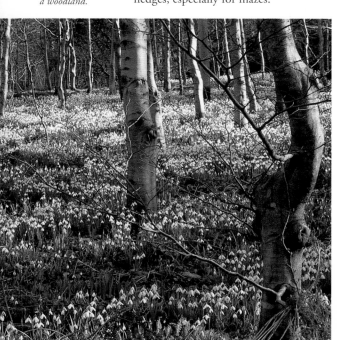

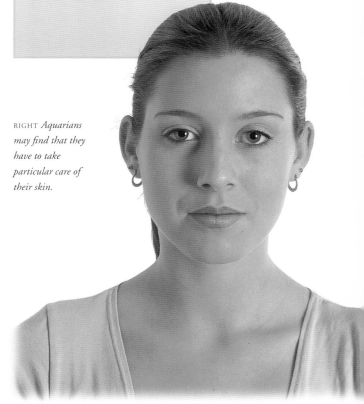

RIGHT *Aquarians may find that they have to take particular care of their skin.*

Elder

Elder grows in temperate areas all over the world and has been used by people everywhere for its beneficial medicinal properties and other uses. Its common name is thought to come from the Anglo-Saxon word for kindle, *aeld,* because the stems, which are hollow, were once used as kindling. The ancient Greeks used elder wood to make musical instruments, including pipes and *sambuke,* a kind of harp, which may be the origin of the elder's Latin name, *Sambucus.* It is one of the most beneficial of healing herbs, and almost every part of it has healing properties.

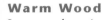

ABOVE Elderberries act as a mild laxative, and with elderflower, they have very warming qualities.

Warm Wood

In some places it was believed that elder wood was warmer to the touch than other woods, because the tree blossoms at the time of the solstice when the sun is at its warmest and most powerful. For this reason, elder wood was often used in henhouses to make shelves and perches, to keep the hens warmer so they would lay better.

Healing with Elder

Elder has a huge number of medicinal uses; it was once known as the "country people's medicine chest" – and probably part of the contents as well as the material for the chest itself! Almost every part of the tree has some use, but most useful are the medicinal flowers and the berries.

The flowers can be used to make elderflower tea, which can be taken for sore throats, coughs, colds, tonsillitis, and as a mild laxative. Elderflower tea is also said to alleviate gout and rheumatism. Elderflowers can also be infused to make an eyewash for eye infections and inflammations, and a compress for chilblains in cold weather.

Elderberries act as a mild laxative, and they have the ability to induce a sweat and bring down a fever. The traditional country cordial "elderberry rob" is made by simmering the berries and thickening the mixture with sugar to make a syrup. This serves as a cordial to treat coughs and colds through the winter.

Elderflowers and elderberries have very warming qualities, and the flowers are an excellent treatment for winter seasonal depression. You won't find them fresh, of course, but you can make (or buy) elderflower wine in the summer and drink a glass or two in the winter to lift your spirits.

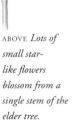

ABOVE Lots of small star-like flowers blossom from a single stem of the elder tree.

Cooking with Elder

Elder is not commonly used as a culinary vegetable, or even a flavoring, but the flowers are occasionally served with fruit, especially gooseberries, or even dipped in batter and deep fried. Both the flowers and the berries are, however, the basis of wine, cordials, champagne, jellies, and jams. The raw flowers taste bitter, but when they are cooked or made into wine, they become mellow and similar in flavor to grapes. The berries are rich in vitamin C, but should not be eaten raw; make sure you cook them at least a little.

ELDERFLOWER CHAMPAGNE

It is the natural yeast in the elderflowers themselves which makes this wine sparkle.

4 ELDERFLOWER HEADS, THE FLOWERS AS FULLY OPEN AS POSSIBLE

1 GALLON (4½ LITERS) COLD WATER

1½ LB. (700G) SUGAR

1 LEMON

2 TBL. WHITE WINE VINEGAR

1 Place some of the water in a double boiler with the sugar and heat until the sugar has dissolved, then cool to room temperature.

2 Squeeze the lemon juice into a large jar or bowl. Cut the rind into three or four pieces and add to the lemon juice.

3 Put the flowerheads into the jar or bowl with the lemon, and add the vinegar.

4 Now pour on the sugar solution and the remaining cold water. Leave this mixture to steep for 4 days.

5 Strain the mixture into airtight bottles and leave for 6 more days.

6 Check the champagne after this time; it may be fizzy enough to drink now or it may need another few days. Serve chilled with ice and lemon.

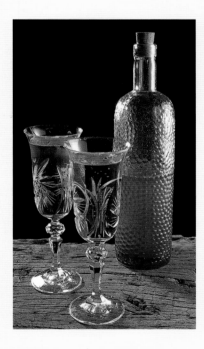

Fumitory

The common and Latin names (*Fumaria officinalis*) of this plant come from the Latin for smoke, perhaps because the wispy leaves look smoky when seen from a distance.

Healing with Fumitory

A cold infusion of fumitory can be applied externally to treat typical Aquarian skin conditions such as dermatitis, eczema, and psoriasis.

Fumitory was used from earliest times to cure all sorts of intestinal problems, especially intestinal obstructions. It was given to both children and horses to expel worms. An infusion drunk as a tea will act as a laxative and a weak diuretic, and can also be used as a general tonic for the digestive system.

SACRED SMOKE

The association of fumitory with smoke led to various strange beliefs, such as the belief that fumitory didn't grow from seeds at all, but emanated from the ground. This may have been due to its smoky appearance. It was also held that if fumitory was burned, its smoke would repel evil spirits.

ABOVE *If burned, it is believed that fumitory will ward off evil spirits.*

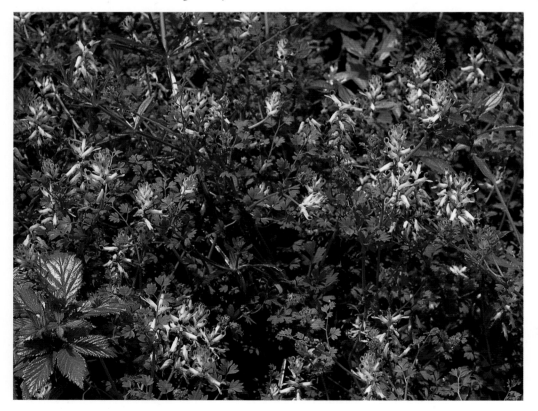

ABOVE *It has been said that the small wispy leaves of fumitory look from a distance like smoke.*

Mullein

This plant has very tall flower spikes, which can reach 7 ft. (2.1m) in height. Its leaves and buds are soft and downy, which makes them function as excellent wicks or tinder.

Roman soldiers used to dip the long, dried stems in tallow to make candles. The texture of the mullein plant, its shape, and its traditional use for burning give it most of its country names, which include "Aaron's rod," "Jacob's staff," "bunny's ears," "Virgin Mary's candle," and "hag's taper."

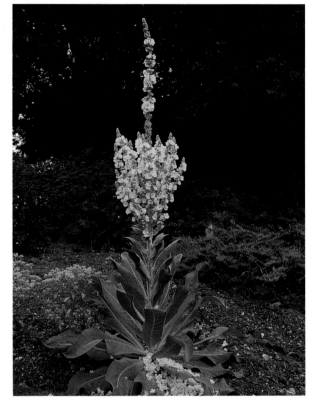

ABOVE *The towering mullein plant has bright yellow candlelike flowers. Legend has it that the Greek hero Odysseus was protected from witches by mullein.*

> **WARNING**
>
> *Apart from the flowers, all other parts of mullein are mildly toxic and should only be taken in small quantities.*

Healing with Mullein

Mullein has long been an important medicinal herb for country folk, who have used it to treat cattle and horses as well as themselves.

One of its chief medicinal uses is for treating colds and respiratory conditions. The flowers can be infused until the water turns yellow, and then drunk to relieve coughs and colds, sore throats, and rhinitis. An infusion of the leaves has much the same effect, but strain it through a fine cloth to remove the hairs, which can be itchy and irritating.

Mullein leaves have been included in smoking mixtures in the past; the dried leaves smoked in a pipe are said to be an effective treatment for ailments of the lungs such as bronchitis and asthma.

Cooking with Mullein

Mullein is not used for cooking, apart from the flowers, which are the nontoxic part of the plant. The flowers are effective for flavoring and coloring liqueurs.

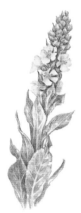

ABOVE *Mullein is toxic apart from the bright yellow flowers which are used as a food colorant.*

> ### MAGICAL HERB
>
> Mullein was considered a magical herb by the ancient people of the Mediterranean. According to Homer, mullein was the herb that was given to Odysseus to protect him from Circe's magic; she turned the rest of his crew into pigs.

Pisces

FEBRUARY 20 – MARCH 20

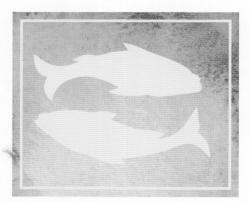

"THESE PEOPLE HAVE A DEEP, HIDDEN LOVE-NATURE, AND ARE ALWAYS ANXIOUS TO GIVE OF THEIR ABUNDANCE TO ALL WHO NEED.... THEY RARELY LOOK FOR DISHONESTY; ON THE CONTRARY, ARE PRONE TO HAVE TOO MUCH CONFIDENCE IN THE WORDS AND PROMISES OF THOSE THEY LOVE."

ELEANOR KIRK *THE INFLUENCE OF THE ZODIAC UPON HUMAN LIFE*

Pisces' traditional ruler is Jupiter, planet of expansion, opportunity, and optimism, although latterday it has been assigned the planet Neptune. The herbs associated with Pisces are rose, lungwort, and meadowsweet.

Before we explore the properties of these herbs, it is worth looking at the herbs that are in season during the cycle of Pisces to discover the role they play in festivals and rituals traditionally held at this time of the year.

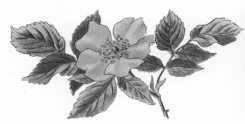
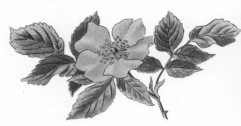

RIGHT *The rose, in all its variety, is associated with the astrological sign of Pisces.*

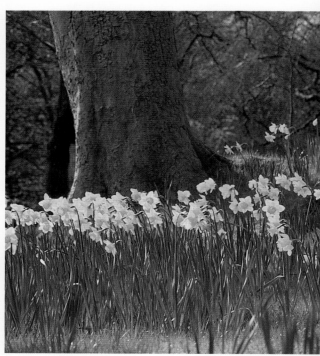

Seasonal Rites

Although none of the major Celtic festivals fall during this period, two important ancient festivals do. The patron saint of Wales, St. David, has his feast day on March 1st; and the Irish patron saint, St. Patrick, is honored on March 17th.

The daffodil is the national flower of Wales because it blooms on St. David's Day. It symbolizes new beginnings because it heralds spring. It is also believed that the day you see the first daffodil open is the time to make a resolution or launch a project.

Lucky Shamrock

St. Patrick's plant is the shamrock, which simply means "little clover." There is some debate over which form of clover is the right one, but the one most often worn by the Irish on St. Patrick's Day is either black medick (*Medicago lupulina*) or Dutch clover (*Trifolium repens*). Whichever clover is chosen, they all have triple leaves, which St. Patrick is said to have used to explain the Holy Trinity.

BELOW *Daffodils are among the flowers that bloom in early Spring. Their golden trumpets herald new beginnings.*

The shamrock is a lucky herb, and the luckiest of all, as everyone knows, is the four-leafed clover. Anyone who owns one of these is immune to cheating and treachery, and everything they undertake will be successful. One St. Patrick's Day ritual is "drowning the shamrock." This entails removing your shamrock from your lapel and putting it in the last drink of the evening (presumably whiskey). When the drink has been downed, the shamrock should be taken from the bottom of the glass and thrown over your left shoulder.

BELOW *Pisceans do not always think to look where they are going and have problems with their feet.*

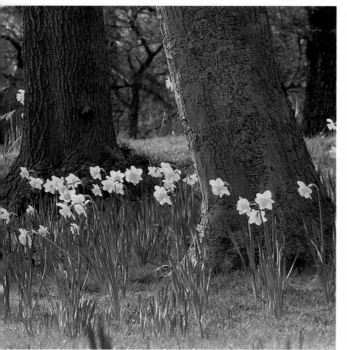

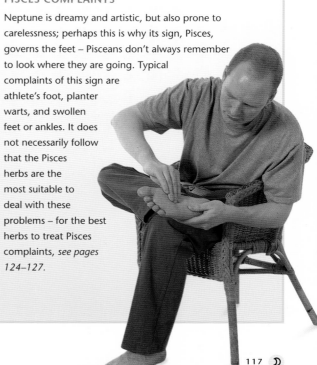

PISCES COMPLAINTS

Neptune is dreamy and artistic, but also prone to carelessness; perhaps this is why its sign, Pisces, governs the feet – Pisceans don't always remember to look where they are going. Typical complaints of this sign are athlete's foot, planter warts, and swollen feet or ankles. It does not necessarily follow that the Pisces herbs are the most suitable to deal with these problems – for the best herbs to treat Pisces complaints, *see pages 124–127.*

Rose

One of the most important herbal flowers of all is ruled by Pisces: the rose. This flower is sacred around the world because of its beauty and scent, and it represents love. The "rose" is sacred to the Virgin Mary in Christian teaching; the word rosary derives from the Latin for "rose garden." The rose is also sacred to the Muslims, and was revered by the ancient Egyptians, Greeks, Romans, and Persians.

Roses and the rosewater derived from them are used for ritual purification. The Hindus anoint themselves with rose oil as a preparation for prayer, and the Muslim leader Saladin, who took Jerusalem, ordered his men to wash the Omar mosque in rosewater to cleanse it.

Healing with Rose

Rose oil is traditionally made from the oldest known cultivated rose, *Rosa gallica officinalis*, also known as the apothecary's rose. The essential oil is widely used in aromatherapy to relax and lift the spirits.

Rose petals are used to make rosewater, which is used in massage oil to cleanse and tone the blood, and to soothe the spirits. Rosewater is an antiseptic tonic for the skin, and is good for treating dry and sore skin. It is also used for splashing on the eyes to help heal conjunctivitis.

The leaves of the rose can be used as a poultice to speed up the healing of wounds, or drunk as a tea that is a tonic and a laxative.

Rose hips are widely used for their health-giving properties; they have an impressive range of valuable ingredients including the vitamins B, E, and K. They are also especially high in vitamin C, the best source being hips from the wild dog rose, *Rosa canina*. The most popular ways of using rose hips are to infuse them as a tea or to make rose hip syrup.

ABOVE *The wild, or "dog," rose has a delicate pink color, and grows in hedges and woodland.*

BELOW *Rosewater makes an ideal tonic for dry or sore skin.*

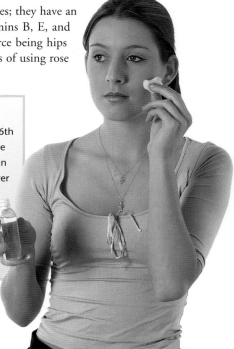

IN SECRET

According to Roman mythology, Cupid consecrated the rose to the god of silence as a bribe, to persuade him to keep quiet about the love affairs of the goddess Venus. This is the origin of the term *sub rosa*, meaning "in secret."

A rose hung above a table, or a plaster rose on the ceiling of a meeting room, was a reminder that everything discussed beneath it was in confidence. In the 16th century, plaster or wooden roses were placed above confessional boxes as an indication that their secrets would never be revealed by a priest, and after 1746 Jacobites could only voice their support for Scotland's Bonnie Prince Charlie *sub rosa*, in the confessional box.

Cooking with Rose

Rose hips have a sharp, bitter taste that is very pleasant when sweetened. You need to remove the fine hairs from the outside, and then use the hips to make jam. Alternatively, purée the rose hips, mix them with honey and lemon juice, and serve as a sauce with red meat such as baked lamb.

Rose flowers are scented and taste sweet, as long as you remove the white heel of the petal, which is bitter. You can sprinkle the leaves over salads or cold desserts, or use them to flavor jam, sorbet, summer drinks, or even vinegar.

TURKISH DELIGHT

1 OZ. (30G) LEAF GELATIN

1 ORANGE

1 LEMON

1 LB. (450G) LOAF SUGAR

⅔ CUP (150ML) ROSEWATER

1 TBL. WHITE RUM

½ CUP (50G) SHELLED PISTACHIOS, BLANCHED AND ROUGHLY CHOPPED

2 CUPS (225G) CONFECTIONER'S SUGAR

1 Soak the leaf gelatine in cold water, according to the instructions on the envelope.

2 Grate the rind of the orange and the lemon finely, and place in a pan. Squeeze the juice from the orange and lemon and strain into the pan.

3 Add the loaf sugar and the rosewater, then bring to a boil.

4 Reduce to a simmer, add the gelatin, and continue to simmer until it is dissolved.

5 Strain the mixture into a large bowl and add the rum. Leave it until it is on the point of setting.

6 Now stir in the pistachios, and pour the mixture into a round dampened cake pan.

7 When the Turkish delight is set, cut it into 1-in. (2.5cm) squares and roll each piece in the sugar.

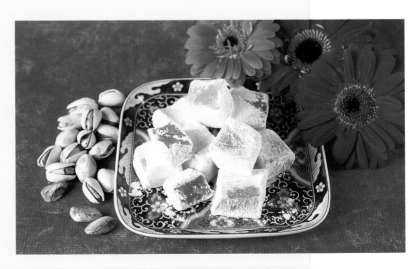

Lungwort

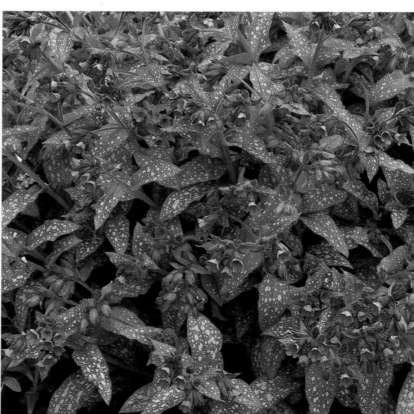

Lungwort derives its name from the fact that the markings on its leaves were thought to resemble the lungs. This also explains its Latin name, *Pulmonaria officinalis,* from the Latin *pulmo* meaning "a lung" *(officinalis* as the second part of a Latin name indicates that the plant was used medicinally). According to the doctrine of signatures, if the plant resembled the lungs, it must be able to cure lung complaints – and it does.

Less prosaically, the white spots on the leaves were said to be drops of milk from the Virgin Mary (which led to a belief that it would be sacrilegious to weed up the plant), or the tears of the Virgin shed after the crucifixion. So lungwort has acquired many country names, such as "Lady's milk," "Good Friday plant," "Lady Mary's tears," "spotted Mary," "Virgin Mary's milkdrops," and "Virgin Mary's tears."

ABOVE *Lungwort is most easily identified by the white spots on its leaves.*

RIGHT *Legend has it that the white spots on the leaves of Lungwort were drops of milk from the breasts of the Virgin Mary.*

RIGHT *Although lungwort is more commonly used for treating chesty coughs and shallow breathing, it can also be added to a poultice for cuts and wounds.*

Healing with Lungwort

Lungwort is true to its name medicinally and is traditionally used to treat respiratory ailments. An infusion of the leaves is a mild expectorant and is used to treat bronchial catarrh, chesty coughs, and shortness of breath. The leaves contain silica, which helps to restore elasticity to the lungs.

Applied externally as a poultice, lungwort leaves are useful for treating minor cuts and wounds.

Lungwort tea has also been used by herbalists to treat diarrhea, hemorrhoids, and gastrointestinal complaints.

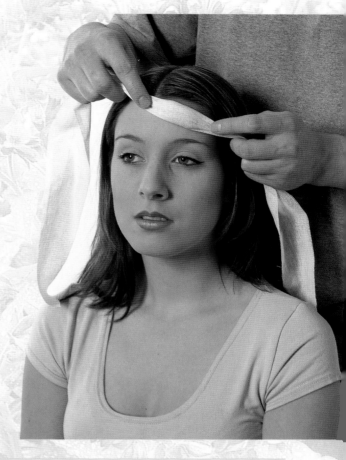

FIGHTING A FEVER

Lungwort is very popular as a herbal treatment to bring down a fever. Try the following recipe:

1 TSP. FRESH LUNGWORT LEAVES

1 TSP. FRESH BORAGE LEAVES

1 TSP. FRESH SORREL LEAVES

½ TSP. GROUND ALLSPICE

2½ CUPS (500ML) BOILING WATER

½ TSP. DARK BROWN SUGAR

1 Infuse the herbs and allspice in the boiling water for about 10 minutes.

2 Add the sugar to sweeten it, and take a small glassful every 2–3 hours.

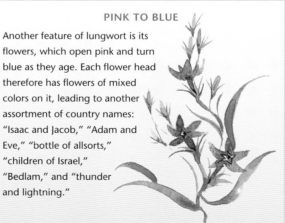

PINK TO BLUE

Another feature of lungwort is its flowers, which open pink and turn blue as they age. Each flower head therefore has flowers of mixed colors on it, leading to another assortment of country names: "Isaac and Jacob," "Adam and Eve," "bottle of allsorts," "children of Israel," "Bedlam," and "thunder and lightning."

Meadowsweet

"Queen of the meadow" is the country name of this herb, which smells strong and sweet, somewhat like hawthorn blossom. Its strong scent gave rise to numerous folk beliefs, such as that smelling it too deeply would send you into a sleep from which you might never awake.

Healing with Meadowsweet

Meadowsweet sap contains salicylic acid, a key ingredient of aspirin. The scientist who first identified this acid produced it from meadowsweet flowers, as well as from the bark of willow (*Salix*), from which it gets its name. In 1899, the drug company Bayer formulated a new drug using this chemical and named it after the old Latin name for meadowsweet, *Spirea ulmaria*: they called it "aspirin."

A tea made by infusing meadowsweet flowers is a mild sedative and painkiller. It is also used to treat heartburn, acid stomach, and peptic ulcers, and also rheumatism and arthritis. Meadowsweet tea is also taken for flu and feverish colds. The dried root can be infused as a treatment for diarrhea.

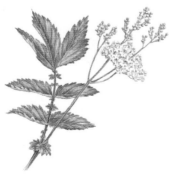

RIGHT *The unassuming white flowers of meadowsweet have a distinctive and powerful aroma.*

Cooking with Meadowsweet

Meadowsweet flowers have a mild nutty flavor, which is often used as a flavoring. Meadowsweet vinegar adds an unusual and pleasant taste to salad dressings and sauces, and the flowers can also be used to flavor jams. They can even be coated in batter and made into fritters – try them combined with elderflowers.

The chief culinary use for meadowsweet, however, has always been as an ingredient in mead and beer. (Mead is a drink made using fermented honey.) The name "medeswete" is thought to be derived not from the word "meadow," as you might suppose, but from the Anglo-Saxon "meadowsweet" because the flowers were used to sweeten mead. If you make your own beer or mead, you could try flavoring it with meadowsweet flowers or leaves, or you can make meadowsweet wine.

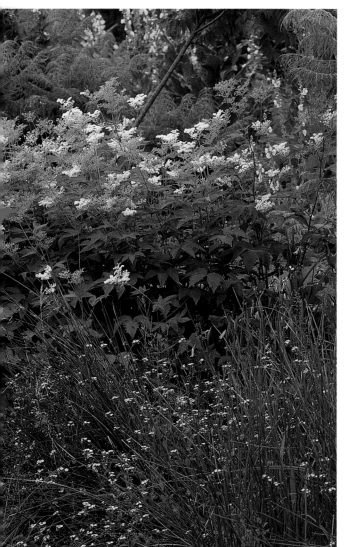

MIXED VIEWS

Like many heavily scented flowers, such as violas and lilies, meadowsweet is often associated with death, and it is considered unlucky by some people to bring it indoors. This is not the prevailing view, however, since meadowsweet has been a popular strewing herb; it was Queen Elizabeth I's favorite. It was also commonly used for strewing churches for weddings and for making bridal bouquets and garlands, which gave rise to another country name: "bridewort."

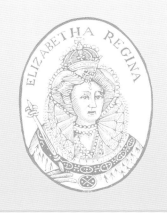

LEFT *Queen Elizabeth I of England was fond of the strewing herb meadowsweet.*

Treating Zodiac-related Symptoms

The following herbs can help with specific zodiac-related symptoms, but of course, for any complaint that might be serious, you should always see a qualified medical practitioner.

HERBS FOR TREATING ARIES COMPLAINTS

COMPLAINT	HERB
Headaches and migraines	feverfew, camomile
Sinuses	golden seal (use small doses only)
Ears	garlic, mullein
Eyes	eyebright, marigold
Hair	rosemary, southernwood

HERBS FOR TREATING TAURUS COMPLAINTS

COMPLAINT	HERB
Sore throat	sage
Tonsillitis	echinacea, thyme
Laryngitis	sage
Coughs	marshmallow, coltsfoot

HERBS FOR TREATING GEMINI COMPLAINTS

COMPLAINT	HERB
Bronchitis	coltsfoot, elecampane, marshmallow
Asthma	coltsfoot, borage
Colds	elderflower, peppermint, garlic
Warts	dandelion, garlic
Chilblains	wolf's bane (arnica)

HERBS FOR TREATING CANCER COMPLAINTS

COMPLAINT	HERB
Premenstrual syndrome	evening primrose
Menstrual problems – painful cramps	raspberry leaf
Menstrual problems – excessive bleeding	agrimony, raspberry leaves
Menstrual problems – absent periods	motherwort, mugwort
Childbirth	raspberry leaf
Breast feeding	vervain, borage, dill, fennel
Menopause	motherwort

HERBS FOR TREATING LEO COMPLAINTS

COMPLAINT	HERB
Varicose veins	horsetail, nettle, St. John's wort
Hemorrhoids	horsetail, pilewort, witch hazel
High blood pressure	garlic
Low blood pressure	broom
Anemia	parsley, nettle
Poor circulation	angelica, juniper

HERBS FOR TREATING VIRGO PROBLEMS

COMPLAINT	HERB
Indigestion	fennel, dill, mint
Nausea	ginger, coriander
Ulcers	licorice, slippery elm
Colitis and IBS (Irritable Bowel Syndrome)	marshmallow root, comfrey root
Constipation	licorice, dandelion root
Diarrhea	agrimony
Diverticulosis	licorice, peppermint

HERBS FOR TREATING LIBRA COMPLAINTS

COMPLAINT	HERB
Cystitis	marshmallow root, horsetail, cranberry juice
Kidney stones	marshmallow root, gravel root (Joe-pye weed)
Enlarged prostate	pumpkin seeds, horsetail, juniper
Bedwetting	horsetail, St. John's wort

HERBS FOR TREATING SCORPIO COMPLAINTS

COMPLAINT	HERB
Impotence	ginseng
Low libido	ginseng, fenugreek, jasmine
Male Low fertility	ginseng, pumpkin seeds
Genitourinary ailments	slippery elm, witch hazel

HERBS FOR TREATING SAGITTARIUS COMPLAINTS

COMPLAINT	HERB
Liver problems	dandelion root, barberry
Gall bladder complaints	dandelion, marshmallow root
Gallstones	dandelion, greater celandine

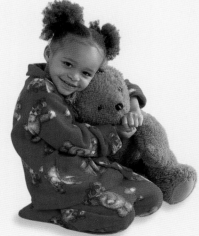

HERBS FOR TREATING CAPRICORN COMPLAINTS

COMPLAINT	HERB
Arthritis	bogbean, devil's claw
Osteoporosis	horsetail, comfrey
Backache	crampbark, wintergreen oil

HERBS FOR TREATING AQUARIUS COMPLAINTS

COMPLAINT	HERB
Acne	evening primrose, rose hip, pumpkin seeds
Spots and boils	echinacea, slippery elm
Psoriasis	red clover, figwort
Eczema	camomile, evening primrose

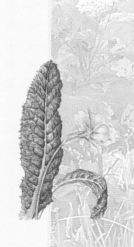

HERBS FOR TREATING PISCES COMPLAINTS

COMPLAINT	HERB
Swollen feet or ankles	oak bark, wormwood
Tired feet	peppermint, rosemary, lavender
Athlete's foot	wild clover
Verrucas	dandelion, garlic
Cold feet (due to poor circulation)	angelica, juniper

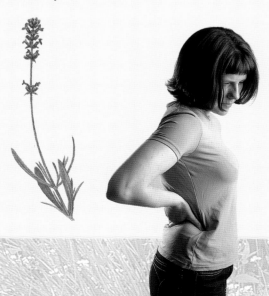

Index

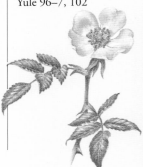